Gynecologic Malignancies

Guest Editor

ORA ISRAEL, MD

PET CLINICS

www.pet.theclinics.com

Consulting Editor
ABASS ALAVI, MD, PhD (Hon), DSc (Hon)

October 2010 • Volume 5 • Number 4

SAUNDERS an imprint of ELSEVIER, Inc.

W.B. SAUNDERS COMPANY
A Division of Elsevier Inc.

1600 John F. Kennedy Boulevard • Suite 1800 • Philadelphia, Pennsylvania 19103-2899

http://www.theclinics.com

PET CLINICS Volume 5, Number 4
October 2010 ISSN 1556-8598, ISBN-13: 978-1-4377-2593-3

Editor: Barton Dudlick
Developmental Editor: Natalie Whitted

PET Clinics (ISSN 1556-8598) is published quarterly by Elsevier Inc., 360 Park Avenue South, New York, NY 10010-1710. Months of issue are January, April, July, and October. Periodicals postage paid at New York, NY, and additional mailing offices. Subscription prices per year are $199.00 (US individuals), $279.00 (US institutions), $102.00 (US students), $226.00 (Canadian individuals), $312.00 (Canadian institutions), $124.00 (Canadian students), $241.00 (foreign individuals), $312.00 (foreign institutions), and $124.00 (foreign students). To receive student and resident rate, orders must be accompanied by name of affiliated institution, date of term, and the signature of program/residency coordinator on institution letterhead. Orders will be billed at individual rate until proof of status is received. Foreign air speed delivery is included in all Clinics subscription prices. All prices are subject to change without notice. POSTMASTER: Send address changes to PET Clinics, Elsevier Health Sciences Division, Subscription Customer Service, 3251 Riverport Lane, Maryland Heights, MO 63043. **Customer Service: 1-800-654-2452 (U.S. and Canada); 314-447-8871 (outside U.S. and Canada). Fax: 314-447-8029. E-mail: journalscustomerservice-usa@elsevier.com (for print support); journalsonlinesupport-usa@elsevier.com (for online support).**

Reprints. For copies of 100 or more of articles in this publication, please contact the Commercial Reprints Department, Elsevier Inc., 360 Park Avenue South, New York, NY 10010-1710. Tel.: 212-633-3812; Fax: 212-462-1935; E-mail: reprints@elsevier.com.

Printed and bound in the United Kingdom
Transferred to Digital Print 2011

Contributors

CONSULTING EDITOR

ABASS ALAVI, MD, PhD (Hon), DSc (Hon)
Professor of Radiology, Division of Nuclear
Medicine, University of Pennsylvania School
of Medicine, Philadelphia, Pennsylvania

GUEST EDITOR

ORA ISRAEL, MD
Head, Department of Nuclear Medicine,
Rambam Health Care Campus; Professor of
Imaging, B. and R. Rappaport Faculty of
Medicine, Technion - Israel Institute of
Technology, Haifa, Israel

AUTHORS

ABASS ALAVI, MD, PhD (Hon) DSc (Hon)
Professor of Radiology, Division of Nuclear
Medicine, University of Pennsylvania School
of Medicine, Philadelphia, Pennsylvania

AMNON AMIT, MD
Division of Gyneco-oncology, Rambam Health
Care Campus, Faculty of Medicine,
Technion-Israel Institute of Technology,
Haifa, Israel

**SANDIP BASU, MBBS (Hons), DRM,
DNB, MNAMS**
Radiation Medicine Centre (BARC), Tata
Memorial Hospital Annexe, Parel, Mumbai, India

DANIEL J. BELL, MBChB
Fellow in Body Imaging, Department of
Radiology, Memorial Sloan-Kettering Cancer
Center, New York City, New York

PRIYA BHOSALE, MD
Department of Diagnostic Radiology,
University of Texas MD Anderson Cancer
Center, Houston, Texas

ROBERT BRISTOW, MD
Divisions of Gynecologic Oncology and
Oncology, Johns Hopkins University School
of Medicine, Baltimore, Maryland

HEDIEH ESLAMY, MD
Division of Nuclear Medicine, Johns Hopkins
University School of Medicine, Baltimore,
Maryland

EINAT EVEN-SAPIR, MD, PhD
Professor, Department of Nuclear Medicine,
Tel Aviv Sourasky Medical Center, Sackler
School of Medicine, Tel-Aviv University,
Tel Aviv, Israel

PERRY W. GRIGSBY, MD
Professor of Radiation Oncology, Nuclear
Medicine and Gynecologic Oncology; Director,
Brachytherapy and MicroRT Treatment Center,
Mallinckrodt Institute of Radiology,
Washington University School of Medicine,
St.Louis, Missouri

ELESYIA D. HAYNES-OUTLAW, MD
Assistant Professor, Department of Radiation
Oncology, University of Texas Southwestern
Medical Center, Dallas, Texas

REVATHY IYER, MD
Department of Diagnostic Radiology,
University of Texas MD Anderson Cancer
Center, Houston, Texas

MEHRBOD SOM JAVADI, MD
Division of Nuclear Medicine, Johns Hopkins
University School of Medicine, Baltimore,
Maryland

ANUJA JHINGRAN, MD
Department of Radiation Oncology Treatment,
University of Texas MD Anderson Cancer
Center, Houston, Texas

THOMAS C. KWEE, MD
Department of Radiology, University Medical
Center Utrecht, Utrecht, The Netherlands

LIOR LOWENSTEIN, MD, MS
Division of Gyneco-oncology, Rambam
Health Care Campus, Faculty of Medicine,
Technion-Israel Institute of Technology,
Haifa, Israel

HARPREET K. PANNU, MD
Associate Attending, Department of
Radiology, Memorial Sloan-Kettering Cancer
Center, New York City, New York

DONALD PODOLOFF, MD
Department of Nuclear Medicine, University
of Texas MD Anderson Cancer Center,
Houston, Texas

ARI REISS, MD
Division of Gyneco-oncology, Rambam Health
Care Campus, Faculty of Medicine,
Technion-Israel Institute of Technology,
Haifa, Israel

JULIAN SCHINK, MD
John I. Brewer Trophoblastic Disease Center,
Northwestern University Feinberg School
of Medicine, Chicago, Illinois

ADITI SHRUTI, MD
Division of Nuclear Medicine, Johns Hopkins
University School of Medicine, Baltimore,
Maryland

RICHARD L. WAHL, MD
Divisions of Nuclear Medicine and Oncology,
Johns Hopkins University School of Medicine,
Baltimore, Maryland

Contents

This article briefly reviews the epidemiology, diagnosis, and treatment of the common gynecologic malignancies, with an emphasis on the shortcomings of current clinical practice. The persistent need to achieve early diagnosis, adjust proper treatment, enhance surveillance, and improve the outcome of these patients has led to the development of new diagnostic modalities. Novel tools such as 18F-fluorodeoxyglucose PET/CT should aim at enhancing the clinician's ability to make critical decisions in treating difficult scenarios.

Patients with gynecologic malignancies are evaluated with a combination of imaging modalities including ultrasonography (US), computed tomography (CT), and magnetic resonance (MR) imaging. US has a primary role in detecting and characterizing endometrial and adnexal pathology. CT is one of the primary modalities in staging malignancy and detecting recurrence. MR imaging is characterized by superior contrast resolution and specificity. This article reviews the role of radiologic imaging for the characterization of gynecologic masses and for staging, planning, and monitoring treatment, as well as for the assessment of tumor recurrence of the most common gynecologic malignancies.

This article summarizes the normal biodistribution of ^{18}F fluorodeoxyglucose in the pelvis, physiologic changes in the female reproductive system and benign adnexal and uterine lesions which may be associated with increased tracer uptake that should be appreciated when PET/CT studies of female patients, mainly those with gynecologic malignancies are reviewed.

Routine screening has lead to significant improvement in the incidence and mortality of cervical cancer in industrialized nations. Current International Federation of Gynecologists and Obstetricians staging is based mainly on clinical examination, with anatomic conventional imaging modalities, such as CT and MR imaging, also being routinely used. Metabolic imaging using 18F-fluoro-2-deoxy-D-glucose(FDG)-PET provides highly specific, noninvasive pretreatment staging and prognostic information regarding post-therapy, and can detect asymptomatic, potentially curable locoregional recurrences. FDG-PET/CT can also optimize the use of advanced radiation treatment planning techniques, such as image-guided intensity modulated radiation therapy, for cervical cancer and may be of value in the development of additional novel approaches, such as stereotactic body radiation therapy.

PET Clinics

THE CLINICS ARE NOW AVAILABLE ONLINE!

Access your subscription at:
www.theclinics.com

GOAL STATEMENT

The goal of the *PET Clinics* is to keep practicing radiologists and radiology residents up to date with current clinical practice in positron emission tomography by providing timely articles reviewing the state of the art in patient care.

ACCREDITATION

PET Clinics is planned and implemented in accordance with the Essential Areas and Policies of the Accreditation Council for Continuing Medical Education (ACCME) through the joint sponsorship of the University of Virginia School of Medicine and Elsevier. The University of Virginia School of Medicine is accredited by the ACCME to provide continuing medical education for physicians.

The University of Virginia School of Medicine designates this educational activity for a maximum of 15 *AMA PRA Category 1 Credits*™ for each issue, 60 credits per year. Physicians should only claim credit commensurate with the extent of their participation in the activity.

The American Medical Association has determined that physicians not licensed in the US who participate in this CME activity are eligible for a maximum of 15 *AMA PRA Category 1 Credits*™ for each issue, 60 credits per year.

Category 1 credit can be earned by reading the text material, taking the CME examination online at http://www.theclinics.com/home/cme, and completing the evaluation. After taking the test, you will be required to review any and all incorrect answers. Following completion of the test and evaluation, your credit will be awarded and you may print your certificate.

FACULTY DISCLOSURE/CONFLICT OF INTEREST

The University of Virginia School of Medicine, as an ACCME accredited provider, endorses and strives to comply with the Accreditation Council for Continuing Medical Education (ACCME) Standards of Commercial Support, Commonwealth of Virginia statutes, University of Virginia policies and procedures, and associated federal and private regulations and guidelines on the need for disclosure and monitoring of proprietary and financial interests that may affect the scientific integrity and balance of content delivered in continuing medical education activities under our auspices.

The University of Virginia School of Medicine requires that all CME activities accredited through this institution be developed independently and be scientifically rigorous, balanced and objective in the presentation/discussion of its content, theories and practices.

All authors/editors participating in an accredited CME activity are expected to disclose to the readers relevant financial relationships with commercial entities occurring within the past 12 months (such as grants or research support, employee, consultant, stock holder, member of speakers bureau, etc.). The University of Virginia School of Medicine will employ appropriate mechanisms to resolve potential conflicts of interest to maintain the standards of fair and balanced education to the reader. Questions about specific strategies can be directed to the Office of Continuing Medical Education, University of Virginia School of Medicine, Charlottesville, Virginia.

The faculty and staff of the University of Virginia Office of Continuing Medical Education have no financial affiliations to disclose.

The authors/editors listed below have identified no professional or financial affiliations for themselves or their spouse/partner:
Abass Alavi, MD (Consulting Editor); Amnon Amit, MD; Sandip Basu, MBBS (Hons), DRM, DNB, MNAMS; Daniel J. Bell, MBChB; Priya Bhosale, MD; Robert Bristow, MD; Barton Dudlick (Acquisitions Editor); Hedieh Eslamy, MD; Einat Even-Sapir, MD, PhD; Perry W. Grigsby, MD; Elesyia Haynes-Outlaw, MD; Revathy Iyer, MD; Mehrbod Som Javadi, MD; Anuja Jhingran, MD; Thomas C. Kwee, MD; Lior Lowenstein, MD, MS; Harpreet K. Pannu, MD; Donald Podoloff, MD; Patrice Rehm, MD (Test Author); Ari Reiss, MD; Julian Schink, MD; and Aditi Shruti, MD.

The authors/editors listed below identified the following professional or financial affiliations for themselves or their spouse/partner:
Ora Israel, MD (Guest Editor) is a consultant for GE Healthcare and an industry funded research/investigator for UltraSPECT.
Richard L. Wahl, MD is on the Advisory Committee/Board for Nihon Medi-Physics, is an industry funded research/investigator for Cellpoint and Molecular Insight Pharmaceutical, and is a consultant for GSK.

Disclosure of Discussion of Non-FDA Approved Uses for Pharmaceutical Products and/or Medical Devices.
The University of Virginia School of Medicine, as an ACCME provider, requires that all faculty presenters identify and disclose any off-label uses for pharmaceutical and medical device products. The University of Virginia School of Medicine recommends that each physician fully review all the available data on new products or procedures prior to clinical use.

TO ENROLL

To enroll in the PET Clinics Continuing Medical Education program, call customer service at 1-800-654-2452 or visit us online at www.theclinics.com/home/cme. The CME program is available to subscribers for an additional fee of $196.00.

Preface
Gynecologic Malignancies

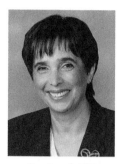

Ora Israel, MD
Guest Editor

Gynecologic malignancies are a widely discussed medical topic in numerous basic research and clinical publications, with respect to their diagnosis, treatment options, and prognosis. These cancers represent a major health care problem worldwide. In the United States alone over 200,000 patients were expected to present with gynecologic malignancies and to account for over 28,000 deaths in 2009. Providing the proper care for patients with gynecologic malignancies is a clinical challenge. There is a need to achieve early diagnosis, decide on the most appropriate treatment strategy, and provide optimal, and as much as possible, noninvasive surveillance, ultimately aiming at improved patient outcome.

New diagnostic modalities have been developed; breakthrough treatment options have been discovered and evaluated in clinical trials. The concept of using metabolic imaging procedures as in vivo indices of the presence and extent of active malignancy, for monitoring the success or resistance to treatment, as well as for early diagnosis of recurrence has evolved over the last few decades and encompasses various types of cancer originating in various organs. Following decades when CT and to a lesser extent ultrasound or MRI were considered the mainstay of noninvasive assessment of gynecologic cancers, the incremental value of the metabolic information provided by PET, mainly using FDG, is now clearly proved. Furthermore, the availability of both metabolic and structural information on single PET/CT studies has made a significant contribution to the understanding of the advantages and limitations of each set of data in the assessment of gynecologic malignancies, to the synergistic value of hybrid imaging subsequently making this technology the diagnostic and treatment-planning modality of choice with proven impact on individual patient care. Hybrid PET/CT using FDG has been almost unconditionally accepted by the imaging community as well as by the referring clinicians as a primary workup tool in patients with gynecologic malignancies.

This issue of *PET Clinics* includes articles from an international multidisciplinary panel of experts. They present a review of the current state-of-the-art knowledge and accepted guidelines for imaging and clinical management of gynecologic malignancies. To all these contributors I extend my heartfelt thanks for their hard work and commitment.

As I have learned from the past, in a professional career that extends over more than three decades, it may be expected that most of the new data presented by our esteemed group of expert contributors in this current issue will be tomorrow's common knowledge or even become obsolete within the next few years. Nevertheless, this issue has been prepared in hope that it will help our present day students be tomorrow's best practitioners and researchers skilled to overcome new challenges.

Ora Israel, MD
Department of Nuclear Medicine
Rambam Health Care Campus
B. and R. Rappaport Faculty of Medicine Technion
- Israel Institute of Technology
6 Ha'Aliya Street
Haifa 35254, Israel

E-mail address:
o_israel@rambam.health.gov.il

PET Clin 5 (2010) ix
doi:10.1016/j.cpet.2010.10.001
1556-8598/10/$ – see front matter

PET/CT in Gynecologic Cancer: Present Applications and Future Prospects—A Clinician's Perspective

Amnon Amit, MD[a],[*], Julian Schink, MD[b], Ari Reiss, MD[a], Lior Lowenstein, MD, MS[a]

KEYWORDS

- ^{18}F-Fluorodeoxyglucose PET • Gynecologic cancer
- Cross-sectional imaging • Best practice

Providing the proper care for patients with gynecologic malignancies has always been a challenge for clinicians. The persistent need to achieve early diagnosis, adjust proper treatment, enhance surveillance, and improve the outcome of these patients has led to the development of new diagnostic modalities. The last decade witnessed great progress in the use of cross-sectional imaging techniques, such as ultrasonography (US), computed tomography (CT), and magnetic resonance (MR) imaging. These imaging modalities are able to demonstrate anatomic details and morphologic changes, but often fail to discriminate between benign and malignant lesions. The functional information obtained from ^{18}F-fluorodeoxyglucose (FDG) PET exhibits the high uptake of glucose by malignant cells, but lacks anatomic landmarks. The fusion of PET with CT combines the advantages of these 2 modalities, allowing the anatomic localization of metabolic abnormalities in the female genital tract and beyond in patients with disseminated disease.

The literature on FDG-PET in gynecologic malignancies between the years 2000 and 2009 reveals a significant increase in the number of articles that have been published. Whereas in 2003 only one article was published, more than 70 articles were listed in 2009, the vast majority reporting on the use of PET/CT. An attempt to obtain similar information concerning CT and MR imaging divulges a constant average number of 90 articles each year. This increase reflects the clinicians' growing interest in this promising modality, which attempts and is often successful in overcoming some limitations of former conventional diagnostic approach.

This article briefly reviews the epidemiology, diagnosis, and treatment of the common gynecologic malignancies, with an emphasis on the shortcomings of current clinical practice.

CERVICAL CANCER
Epidemiology

Cervical cancer is one of the leading causes of death among women with gynecologic malignancies[1] and the median age of diagnosis is approximately 48 years in the United States. Recent studies indicate that human papilloma virus (HPV) infection is the main cause of this disease.[2] High-risk viral subtypes (mainly types 16 and 18) increase the risk of developing high-grade cervical dysplasia and cancer. Important risk factors

[a] Division of Gyneco-oncology, Rambam Health Care Campus, Faculty of Medicine, Technion-Israel Institute of Technology, Haifa 9602, Israel
[b] John I. Brewer Trophoblastic Disease Center, Northwestern University Feinberg School of Medicine, 250 East Superior Street, Suite 5-2168, Chicago, IL, USA
* Corresponding author. Department of Obstetrics and Gynecology, Rambam Medical Center, 9 Ha'Aliya Street, Haifa 31096, Israel.
E-mail address: a_amit@rambam.health.gov.il

PET Clin 5 (2010) 391–405
doi:10.1016/j.cpet.2010.07.001
1556-8598/10/$ – see front matter © 2010 Elsevier Inc. All rights reserved.

include increased number of sexual partners, early age at first coitus, low socioeconomic status, compromised immune system, smoking, and diethylstilbestrol exposure. Most cervical cancers are squamous in histology, with adenocarcinoma being the second most common histologic type.

Prevention and Screening

Two HPV vaccines have recently been approved by the United States Food and Drug Administration. These vaccines were developed against the viral subtypes 16 and 18, which are responsible for 75% of cervical cancers. Recent studies have demonstrated that these vaccines are highly immunogenic and reduce rates of cervical intraepithelial neoplasia significantly, with an efficacy near 100% in women previously not exposed to these viral subtypes. The recommendations from the United States Centers for Disease Control and Prevention and from other medical authorities are to begin vaccination at the age of 11 or even as early as 9 years.[3]

Because invasive cervical cancer has a preinvasive phase (cervical intraepithelial neoplasia), screening is an effective tool in risk reduction. Regular Pap smear screening, as done in the United States, has dramatically reduced the incidence and mortality of this disease. Although sensitivity for a single examination is relatively low (50%–70%), repeat examinations (every 2–3 years) may at least partly overcome this limitation. It has also been suggested that the identification of high-risk types of HPV has improved the sensitivity and specificity of the Pap smear test in certain circumstances, such as when having atypical cells or atypical glandular cells of undetermined significance (ASCUS/AGUS). However, HPV typing as a screening modality has yet to be evaluated, mainly for its cost effectiveness.

Natural Course of the Disease

Following a preinvasive stage, located mainly in the squamo-columnar junction, the cancer invades the cervical stroma and then spreads by direct invasion into the parametrium, uterus, and vagina. As the disease advances, the tumor spreads through lymphatic channels toward the pelvic, para-aortic, and supraclavicular lymph nodes. Hematogenic spread to the lungs, liver, or any other distant organ may be observed at any stage, although it is unlikely to occur in the early stages of the disease.

Diagnosis

Following an abnormal Pap test, women are evaluated with colposcopy and directed biopsies. In the case of high-grade intraepithelial lesions (HGSIL) or in cases of suspected pathologic Pap smear along with suboptimal colposcopy, conization of the cervix is recommended.

Staging

In contrast to endometrial and ovarian cancer, cervical cancer is staged clinically, because of the prevalence of the disease in underserved countries where technology is not available. **Table 1** summarizes the International Federation for Gynecology and Obstetrics (FIGO) clinical staging, treatment options, and 5-year survival

Table 1
FIGO clinical staging, treatment, and 5-year survival for cervical cancer

FIGO Stage Criteria	Treatment Options	5-Year Survival
O. Carcinoma in situ	Conization, TAH	96%–100%
IA. Microscopic lesions	Conization, modified hysterectomy[a]	92%–94%
IB1. Macroscopic lesion ≤4 cm	RH, RTL, XRT/Chemo	80.7%
IB2. Macroscopic lesion ≥4 cm	RH, XRT/Chemo	79%
IIA. Vaginal involvement	RH, XRT/Chemo	76%
IIB. Parametrial involvement	XRT/Chemo	73.3%
IIIA. Lower one-third of vagina	XRT/Chemo	50.5%
IIIB. Side wall extension and/or hydronephrosis	XRT/Chemo	46%
IVA. Adjacent organ involvement	XRT/Chemo	29%
IVB. Distant metastasis	Chemo, palliative XRT	22%

Abbreviations: Chemo, chemotherapy; RH, radical hysterectomy; RTL, radical trachelectomy; TAH, total abdominal hysterectomy; XRT, radiotherapy.
[a] Individualization by patient's age and fertility desire.

rates for every stage. Staging procedures include physical examination, chest radiograph, intravenous pyelogram (IVP), cystoscopy, and rectoscopy. However, most medical centers employ cross-sectional imaging techniques such as US, CT, MR imaging, and FDG-PET/CT to overcome the limitations of traditional diagnostic methods. Surgical staging with lymphadenectomy is more accurate than clinical staging, but is controversial among gynecologic oncologists, as there is no proof of any survival benefits of the procedure, especially with microscopic nodal disease.[4] Using new diagnostic modalities or any information obtained from surgical procedures will not change staging, but may lead to treatment adjustment.

Treatment

Treatment in the early stages of the disease includes surgery or radiotherapy. In locally advanced disease, radiotherapy is combined with chemotherapy, and in metastatic disease the treatment is chemotherapy.[5–7] Patients with early (Stage IA) squamous cell cancer (microinvasive) and no lymph-vascular space invasion (LVSI) can be treated with simple, extrafascial hysterectomy. Stage IB to IIA disease is usually treated with radical hysterectomy and pelvic lymphadenectomy, but can be treated with primary radiation therapy with similar outcomes.[8] However, clinicians and patients alike tend to opt for surgery because of the possible complications of radiation, including loss of ovarian function, bowel stricture, and fistula formation.

Young females with early disease desiring future fertility can be treated with conization of the cervix alone or with radical trachalectomy, which removes the cervix, parametrial tissue, and upper vagina while preserving the uterus for future childbearing. A permanent cervical cerclage and assisted reproductive technologies are required in this setting. Prognosis appears to be acceptable in this group regarding survival, recurrence, and pregnancy outcomes. However, these patients need close follow-up so as to exclude recurrence.[4,9]

When the cancer has progressed beyond the cervix, but is still limited to the pelvis (Stages IIB through IVA), primary chemo-radiotherapy is used. Radiation therapy is delivered by a combination of tele- and brachytherapy to deliver an adequate dose to the cervix, parametrium, and pelvic lymph nodes. Hysterectomy may be performed after radiation therapy in patients with residual disease. However, the morbidity caused by combining surgery and chemo-radiotherapy must be taken into consideration in such cases.

Postoperative chemo-radiotherapy is recommended for patients who have had a radical hysterectomy with the following risk factors for final pathology: parametrial involvement, close or positive vaginal margins, positive lymph nodes, and certain tumor characteristics such as LVSI, tumor size, and deep stromal invasion.[7] Distant metastatic cervical cancer (Stage IVB) has a poor prognosis and is palliated with chemotherapy, which provides a limited survival benefit. The combination of cisplatin and topotecan is currently the treatment of choice.[10]

Recurrence

Recurrent cervical cancer has a dismal prognosis if not limited to the pelvis. If the recurrent disease is limited to the central pelvis without other metastases, and if no pelvic side-wall involvement is identified, long-term survival may be achieved. Radiation therapy is recommended for locally confined recurrent disease in patients who have not already undergone this treatment. In previously radiated patients, pelvic exenteration (anterior, posterior, or total) offers survival rates of 20% to 60%.[11] With nonresectable disease, overall survival is less than 1 year.

Special Considerations and Unmet Clinical Needs in the Evaluation and Treatment of Patients with Cervical Cancer

This section updates and summarizes the clinician's needs in specific areas.

Staging and evaluation of newly diagnosed patients with cervical cancer

The main challenge in this group of patients is to choose the best treatment in terms of survival benefits with the lowest toxicity. Following initial diagnosis, this group is usually divided into 3 subgroups.

Patients with early disease: Stages I to IIA These patients may be treated by either radical hysterectomy or pelvic radiotherapy, with a similar overall survival. However, many patients who undergo radical hysterectomy are subsequently referred to radiotherapy secondary to failure of clinical and imaging modalities, despite the fact it can result in long-term toxicity with no survival benefits.

All current modalities that are expected to guide surgeons in assessing invasion into the cervical stroma and early parametrial involvement are characterized by a relatively low sensitivity in the early stages of the disease.[12] Clinicians are therefore unable to avoid bimodality treatment. Thus, even though the disease is confined to the cervix, these patients will be referred to radiotherapy to reduce the chances of recurrence.

Another main concern is pelvic and para-aortic lymph node (PALN) status. Positive pelvic lymph nodes are the most important prognostic factor, and radical hysterectomy may be abandoned if suspected positive lymph nodes are detected in frozen-section pathology. FDG-PET/CT, with its high specificity, may allow clinicians to avoid unnecessary surgery and to refer patients to chemo-radiotherapy, making it the imaging procedure of choice in evaluating this group of patients. These patients will be closely followed secondary to a high probability of recurrence.

Semiquantitative measurements of the degree of FDG uptake using maximum standardized uptake value (SUV_{max}) was recently studied in several aspects of cervical cancer. Further experience is needed to estimate the use of this modality in characterizing the aggressiveness of a tumor and in predicting stromal invasion and pelvic lymph node metastasis.[13]

Patients with locally advanced disease These patients represent, according to clinical staging, 15% to 30% of patients with pelvic disease who will eventually have lymph node metastases.[4] Patients with locally advanced disease are usually treated with chemo-radiotherapy. The goal in treating these patients is to exclude extrapelvic disease and to achieve the best definition for a radiation field. Positive PALN may alter the radiation field and lead to a different chemotherapy regimen. Disseminated disease may change the approach of treatment in the direction of palliative care and obviate the need for radiation in end-stage patients.

Several studies have demonstrated the superiority of FDG imaging over CT and MR imaging in detecting metastatic lesions in patients with advanced disease.[14–17] PET/CT provides better localization and definition of metastatic sites.[18] The sensitivity of FDG-PET is in direct correlation with the stage of disease and probably relates to the volume of the tumor present in affected nodes.[19] For patients with advanced disease, the sensitivity of FDG-PET/CT in detecting PALN metastases is 95%.[17,20,21] A limitation of some these studies is that they did not use histopathology as a gold standard, because most patients did not undergo a surgical procedure. Other drawbacks are related to the fact that PET/CT results were not always translated into survival benefits, and also that most studies include a relatively small number of patients. However, the superiority of PET/CT over CT and MR imaging has emerged from many studies in different medical centers.

Assuming that patients with advanced disease will have a worse prognosis, the accuracy of these results is often dependent on a relatively long-term follow-up, which may partially overcome the lack of pathology results. Up-to-date PET/CT results are an indicator of its importance as a tool to be used in evaluating patients with locally advanced disease. Future efforts should focus on improving the accuracy of disease detection through the fusion of PET with another modality, such as MR imaging, or through the use of other metabolic agents.

Patients with metastatic cervical cancer When newly diagnosed, these patients have a poor prognosis (see **Table 1**). Treatment is primarily palliative, with the goal being control of symptoms. Some studies have demonstrated the ability to detect, characterize, and locate lesions in supraclavicular and mediastinal lymph nodes, lungs, bones, peritoneum, omentum, and liver.[22–24] Because metastatic disease in newly diagnosed patients is uncommon, comparative studies demonstrating the additional value of PET/CT are scarce. Clinicians may gain some experience from recurrent studies that enable one to demonstrate the value of PET/CT in restaging these patients and specifically assessing distant lesions.

Radiotherapy planning

Radiotherapy in patients with cervical cancer aims at destroying malignant lesions by delivering maximal doses to a specific location while attempting to avoid the radiation of healthy tissues. Because radiotherapy can cause severe toxicity, there is a true clinical need to define the borders between healthy and malignant tissue in the primary tumor. Having a diagnostic modality that can provide this information can be very helpful for clinicians in their efforts to improve radiotherapy planning and outcome.

As previously noted, PET/CT has been shown to have the best accuracy in detecting disease in lymph nodes and distant lesions, and therefore is the most useful tool for directing radiotherapists to the affected sites. Many recent studies have been conducted using FDG-PET/CT to demonstrate the actively metabolic borders of the primary cervical tumor and distant active lesions. According to these studies, PET/CT images should be transferred to the radiotherapy treatment planning system so that the contour of normal organs can be delivered from the CT portion and metastatic active sites can be contoured from the PET component. Subsequent radiation doses at the prescribed volume can be planned using the radiotherapy treatment planning software.[19] Additional studies need to be conducted in the future to establish the role and integration of PET/CT in radiotherapy treatment planning systems.

Determination of prognostic pretreatment parameters and response to therapy

Assessing a patient's prognosis is of great importance, as it may change treatment planning to improve outcome. Prognosis can be determined by pretreatment parameters and by response to treatment, which may dictate additional therapy and/or a different follow-up policy (see **Table 1**). Before the introduction of PET/CT, prognosis was estimated by the patient's age, stage, grade, presence of positive pelvic and PALN, and by other tumor indices, such as tumor volume and lymph and vascular space involvement.[18]

In many medical centers, PET/CT is now routinely performed for pretreatment evaluation and prognosis determination. Experience gained over the last few years indicates that PET/CT is of additional value in determining the patient's prognosis and treatment response, mainly due to its high accuracy in detecting affected lymph nodes. Moreover, studies have shown that evaluating a patient's prognosis using SUV_{max} values in primary tumors and assessing the metabolic activity 3 months after completion of radiotherapy may provide important information for significantly improving the outcome.[13,25–28] Brooks and colleagues[26] evaluated the role of PET/CT in detecting symptomatic versus asymptomatic recurrent cervical cancer. Their findings demonstrated a significant survival benefit in asymptomatic patients with recurrent disease detected by PET/CT as compared with symptomatic patients.[26] This study and others have led some medical centers to implement PET/CT as a routine diagnostic imaging modality for patients with cervical cancer.

Patient follow-up and early detection of recurrent disease

Surveillance protocols of patients with cervical cancer usually consist of a physical examination, Pap smear, and a chest radiograph performed at different intervals according to risk factors. However, it is uncommon to detect a symptomatic patient using this surveillance policy. Pelvic examination and vaginal or cervical cytology are of limited use because of radiation-associated changes. Obliteration of the vaginal vault is common, and parametrial fibrosis increases the difficulties of assessing the normal anatomy.[29–31] Evaluation of lymph node status using a pelvic examination is impossible, making it highly unlikely

that recurrence of the disease will be detected in asymptomatic patients.

As already noted, the implementation of routine CT scans has not been shown to contribute significantly to outcome. MR imaging shows better results than CT, but is not good enough to be used as a routine imaging modality.[32] Morice and colleagues[33] showed that using CT and MR imaging during routine follow-up did not change the survival rates of patients with cervical cancer. These limitations increase the clinician's need for a better diagnostic modality that allows detection of asymptomatic recurrence. Early detection of central pelvic recurrence may result in salvage surgery (ie, pelvic exenteration) with curative intent and survival benefits.

In summary, FDG-PET/CT meets the clinical need for an effective imaging modality in the early detection of recurrent disease, and provides better localization and definition of metastatic sites in patients with advanced disease. The evidence supports that PET/CT be used for routine follow-up purposes and can provide a better outcome. However, surveillance intervals should be further investigated to define the survival benefits and cost effectiveness.

OVARIAN CANCER
Epidemiology

Ovarian cancer is the sixth most common malignancy in women worldwide and the second most common gynecologic malignancy, accounting for about 21,500 new cases and 15,000 deaths a year in the United States. The lifetime risk of developing ovarian cancer is about 1.6%.[34] Despite strenuous research and screening efforts, this malignancy still constitutes a major diagnostic and therapeutic problem.

Epithelial tumors account for about 90% of malignant ovarian tumors.[35] Less common types are germ cell or stromal tumors. Commonly known risk factors are age, family history, genetics, nulliparity, early menarche, and late menopause.[36] More than two-thirds of ovarian cancers present during the postmenopausal period, at a median age of 63 years.[37] Family history is recognized as a significant risk factor, with women whose mothers had ovarian cancer carrying a 7% risk of developing the disease themselves.[38]

The most common genetic mutations associated with ovarian cancer are BRCA-1 and BRCA-2, commonly found among Ashkenazi Jews. The average cumulative risk for ovarian cancer by age 70 years is 39% (18%–54%) in BRCA-1 mutation carriers and 11% (2.4%–19%) in BRCA-2 mutation carriers. Lynch syndrome (hereditary nonpolyposis colon cancer syndrome) is another genetic entity associated with an increase in the lifetime risk for ovarian cancer of up to 10% to 15%.[39] The use of oral contraceptives,[40] parity, and bilateral oopherectomy are known to be protective factors against the development of ovarian cancer.

Diagnosis

The main challenges of the primary practitioner in the early diagnosis of ovarian cancer are the lack of specific early signs and symptoms and the absence of effective screening programs. About 75% of cases are diagnosed at an advanced stage, leading to high morbidity and poor survival rates.[41,42] Most commonly, the tumor spreads into the peritoneal cavity. Lymphatic and hematogenic spread are less common routes of dissemination for this type of tumor.[43,44]

The majority of patients present with vague and nonspecific symptoms, such as abdominal discomfort and distention. In a more advanced stage patients may present with gastrointestinal symptoms secondary to bowel obstruction. Tumor metastases to liver parenchyma and extra-abdominal organs, as well as pleural effusion, are relatively uncommon and are more characteristic of late stages of the disease.

Diagnosis relies on the detection of pelvic and abdominal masses, and ascites.[45,46] Patients with suspected ovarian cancer undergo a thorough physical examination, including abdominal palpation and bimanual vaginal examination. In most cases, an adnexal mass is palpated. Other abdominal masses may be recognized in advanced cases. Serum levels of CA125 (a glycoprotein tumor marker) can be useful in distinguishing malignant from benign pelvic masses, especially in postmenopausal patients. The combination of an adnexal mass with an elevated serum level of CA125 >200 IU/mL in a postmenopausal woman was found to have a positive predictive value of 97% for ovarian cancer diagnosis.[47–49]

Imaging modalities are commonly used for diagnosing abdominal masses and differentiating them from ovarian cancer. Common sonographic signs related to ovarian cancer are complex ovarian masses, irregular cysts with papillae, low-resistance flow in ovarian blood vessels as measured by Doppler, and ascites.[50] CT is commonly used for the evaluation of disease spread and for the differentiation of ovarian cancer from other malignancies.[51]

Treatment

The standard treatment of ovarian cancer includes cytoreductive surgery and chemotherapy drugs. The goal of surgery is to remove all tumor load, so-called optimal debulking.[52–56] During surgery, a total hysterectomy, bilateral salpingo-oophorectomy, and infracolic omentectomy are performed. Peritoneal biopsies and retroperitoneal lymph node sampling are also performed as part of the staging process.

To obtain optimal debulking, any macroscopically visible tumor needs to be surgically removed.[57,58] The significance of optimal debulking is its association with prognosis of ovarian cancer.[59,60] Patients whose tumor has been completely resected to a state of no macroscopic residual disease are found to have significantly better survival rates than patients who still have remaining macroscopic tumor.[60] In some cases, surgical removal of the entire tumor may not be feasible due to poor patient condition, stage IV disease, or high metastatic tumor load.[61,62]

Neoadjuvant chemotherapy, consisting of 3 to 4 courses of intravenous chemotherapy administered before the surgical procedure, is commonly used to reduce the tumor burden and allow optimal debulking. A recent large prospective, randomized, controlled multicenter study conducted by the gynecologic cancer group (EORTC-GCG) demonstrated that in cases of advanced ovarian tumors, neoadjuvant chemotherapy followed by interval debulking surgery may result in similar survival rates as those for standard primary debulking surgery followed by adjuvant chemotherapy.[63–65] Adjuvant chemotherapy is needed in cases of tumor capsule penetration and beyond. Nowadays, different chemotherapy drugs are used for treating ovarian cancer. Current first-line chemotherapy for epithelial tumors is the combination of paclitexal plus a platinum analogue for 6 to 8 cycles.[66–68] Ongoing research in chemotherapy for ovarian cancer is driven by both drug companies and gyneco-oncologist research groups, such as the gynecologic oncology group (GOG).

Prognosis

Prognosis of ovarian cancer is highly dependent on tumor stage, histologic type and differentiation, surgical outcome (optimal debulking versus nonoptimal debulking), and other comorbidity factors. A study by Heintz and colleagues[69] demonstrated that survival rates are highly associated with the surgical stage of the disease at diagnosis. The approximate 5-year survival rate of patients is: Stage I disease, 90%; Stage II, 65%;

Stage III, 40%; and Stage IV, 18%.[69] Although the overall response rate with primary therapy is about 80%, the majority of patients will ultimately relapse and die of the disease within 5 years of diagnosis.[70,71] If the disease recurs within 6 months following treatment, it is considered to be platinum-resistant. Chemotherapy for platinum-resistant patients includes pegylated and liposomal drugs, doxorubicin, Hycamtin (topotecan hydrochloride), and gemcitabine. A second-look operation is performed for the evaluation of treatment response. Its current use is mainly for research purposes.

Staging

In recent years, FDG-PET/CT has been recognized as a new modality that can potentially assist in the diagnosis of tumor spread and in the detection of early recurrence of the disease.[72–74] Current screening algorithms, using the measurement of CA125 serum levels and ultrasound imaging of the ovaries, have yielded low positive predictive values, and their ability to lower the stage of disease at the time of diagnosis remains questionable.[75] PET/CT might have a potential role in improving the screening algorithms. There are sporadic case reports describing the detection of early-stage ovarian cancer using PET/CT.[76,77] Risum and colleagues[73] suggested the use of PET/CT in cases who present with elevated CA125 serum levels, combined with a suspected ovarian mass seen on US. The sensitivity and specificity of PET/CT in such cases was 100% and 92%, respectively.

Prevention and Screening

Early diagnosis is probably the key point in reducing the mortality and morbidity associated with ovarian cancer. Patients diagnosed at an early stage (Stage I) have a significantly better diagnosis than patients diagnosed at a late stage (Stages III and IV), with 5-year survival rates estimated at 90% and 25%, respectively.[78] Intensive research is currently ongoing to identify additional markers and a cost-effective screening strategy. Several screening programs using ultrasound and CA125 serum levels demonstrated relatively earlier stage detection, but failed to show survival benefits.

Evidence suggests that screening programs are appropriate for women with a family history of ovarian cancer or familial ovarian cancer syndromes. Previous research has evaluated the role of screening programs in the early detection of ovarian cancer in high-risk populations.[79,80] In one study, 4 years of screening with CA125 serum levels and transvaginal ultrasound revealed a sensitivity of 40% and a specificity of 99% in a series of 312 women 35 years or older, and carriers for BRCA-1 or BRCA-2 mutations.[81]

Screening recommendations for higher-risk women depend on whether there is a known or suspected hereditary cancer syndrome. Diagnostic modalities such as CT and MR imaging have been tested and have not demonstrated any advantage in this regard. Many other tumor markers are under investigation, but as yet lack clinical application. The role of PET/CT has not been thoroughly explored, but possible limitations for the use of this modality for screening are its high cost and lack of specificity.

Once the disease has been diagnosed, there is a question regarding the additive role of additional imaging modalities in treatment planning.[74,82] The utility of CT in determining complete resection of the tumor in advanced cases is of limited value.[83] Several studies have investigated the incremental value of preoperative PET/CT to estimate the feasibility of achieving optimal debulking in an advanced disease stage.[74] Previous studies have also demonstrated stage migration when comparing PET/CT with CT.[73] However, PET/CT is still not being routinely used preoperatively for such purposes.

Following the diagnosis of ovarian tumor, preoperative evaluation should be aimed to achieve several objectives:

1. Rule out other primary tumors with metastases to the ovaries (mainly of breast or gastrointestinal origin).
2. Estimate the feasibility of achieving optimal debulking. Once it is determined that complete resection of the tumor is not possible, neoadjuvant treatment may be administered. Although the neoadjuvant approach has not been proven to increase survival rates, it may have a positive impact on quality of life.
3. Gain better knowledge concerning the location of any metastasis to assign the ideal team for surgery (urologist, general surgeon, and so forth).

Recurrence

Patient follow-up and evaluation for recurrence of the disease is done mainly by periodic physical examination, repeated testing of CA125 serum levels, and CT if needed.[84] The add-on value of early detection of disease recurrence is controversial, with recent studies demonstrating that apart from the increase in the number of chemotherapy courses administered, there was no added benefit in terms of survival time and quality of life in cases where early recurrence was detected. Based on these data, it is not clear whether tests with higher sensitivity are clinically effective in the earlier detection of disease recurrence.

When disease recurs, the clinician needs to know whether it is a localized recurrence or disseminated disease. This information is crucial in making the decision to attempt a second debulking. If the disease is disseminated, the clinician needs a reliable method for monitoring treatment results in order to avoid unnecessary chemotherapy if it fails to achieve a response. PET/CT appears to play a potentially important role in early detection of recurrent ovarian cancer and, if detected, in determining whether it is localized or disseminated.

The differentiation between a borderline and a full-blown tumor is also highly significant. A borderline tumor can usually be treated by unilateral oopherectomy. Clinical evaluation and presurgical assessment can assist in better planning of surgery. Neither CT nor US are good tools for differentiating between borderline and malignant tumors. Risum and colleagues[73] have reported normal metabolic results in all their 7 cases diagnosed with borderline tumors.

Other than early primary diagnosis of the disease, early detection of tumor recurrence and the differentiation between borderline and full-blown tumors are among the most common challenging issues in the management of ovarian cancer today. Cumulative research in gynecology is required to determine the role of PET/CT in helping to resolve them.

ENDOMETRIAL CANCER
Epidemiology

Endometrial cancer, a tumor of the endometrial lining of the uterine corpus, is the most common genital tract cancer, and the fourth most common malignancy occurring in women living in developed countries worldwide.[85] This disease trails only breast, colon, and lung cancer, with an estimated 136,000 cases per year. Endometrial cancer is associated with excess estrogen levels, either from endogenous or exogenous sources. Obesity and diabetes are linked to increased levels of circulating unbound endogenous estrogen, and with the epidemic of obesity, the incidence of this cancer is expected to increase.

Background and Natural Course of the Disease

The overall prognosis for endometrial cancer is 75%, with greater than 90% disease-free survival for women with Stage I disease. The good outcome seen in this malignancy reflects that early diagnosis usually occurs when women report abnormal vaginal bleeding, either postmenopausal or heavy intermenstrual bleeding. The tumor is generally confined to the uterus at the time of diagnosis, with only 10% to 20% of surgically staged patients having lymph node metastases at the time of surgery.[85] The staging system for endometrial cancer is defined by FIGO. The recent revision of this staging system in 2009 (**Box 1**), is based on surgical staging that ideally includes total hysterectomy, bilateral salpingo-oophorectomy, pelvic and PALN dissection, and assessment of peritoneal cytology. Lymph node metastases and survival are predicted by depth of myometrial invasion, tumor grade, histology, and tumor size.[86]

Diagnosis and Pretreatment Assessment

The diagnosis of endometrial cancer is usually the result of an office endometrial biopsy or uterine

---

Box 1
Carcinoma of the endometrium

Stage I: Tumor confined to the corpus uteri

  IA: No or less than half myometrial invasion

  IB: Invasion equal to or more than half of the myometrium

Stage II: Tumor invades cervical stroma, but does not extend beyond the uterus

Stage III: Local and/or regional spread of the tumor

  IIIA: Tumor invades the serosa of the corpus uteri and/or adnexae

  IIIB: Vaginal and/or parametrial involvement

  IIIC: Metastases to pelvic and/or para-aortic lymph nodes

    IIIC1: Positive pelvic nodes

    IIIC2: Positive para-aortic lymph nodes with or without positive pelvic lymph nodes

Stage IV: Tumor invades bladder and/or bowel mucosa, and/or distant metastases

  IVA: Tumor invasion of bladder and/or bowel mucosa

  IVB: Distant metastases, including intra-abdominal metastases and/or inguinal lymph nodes

Note: Endocervical glandular involvement only should be considered as Stage I and no longer as Stage II. Positive cytology has to be reported separately without changing the stage.

dilatation and curettage (D&C), with or without hysteroscopy, performed under sedation in a surgical suite. These procedures are indicated if a woman complains of unexplained postmenopausal bleeding, has abnormal glandular cells on her Pap smear, or an ultrasonogram showing a thickened endometrial stripe. Evaluation of postmenopausal bleeding or increased risk of endometrial cancer by US is a noninvasive alternative. Karlsson and colleagues[87] performed a prospective trial of transvaginal US evaluation in 1168 women with postmenopausal bleeding scheduled for D&C. These investigators found that for a US cut-off of 5 mm, no women with a stripe below 5 mm had endometrial cancer. If a postmenopausal woman has an endometrial stripe of 5 mm or greater, then her risk of endometrial cancer is found to be 31%.[88] The 5-mm threshold is only accurate in women who are postmenopausal and not using hormone replacement therapy. The use of US as a noninvasive test for evaluation of postmenopausal women is attractive because it is relatively painless and readily available. A meta-analysis has shown that the 5-mm threshold is 96% sensitive for detecting cancer, but has a 4% false-negative rate and a 50% false-positive rate.[89] The value of this noninvasive evaluation is in ruling out endometrial cancer without performing a biopsy. Ultimately, if the woman has a thickened stripe, then an endometrial biopsy or D&C is indicated before definitive surgery with hysterectomy.

For women diagnosed with endometrial cancer, the routine pretreatment assessment includes a thorough physical examination, laboratory studies, and a chest radiograph. Routine CT or MR imaging are not useful unless the patient is suspected of having metastatic disease.

Pretreatment or Preoperative Evaluation

The risks of lymph node staging in endometrial cancer, combined with the lack of surgical expertise and no proven benefit, invite the use of a noninvasive test that predicts metastatic disease. To date, studies of CT, MR imaging, and FDG imaging have failed to show significant benefit from the use of these modalities in the preoperative evaluation of women scheduled to undergo hysterectomy for endometrial cancer. CT and MR imaging detection of lymph node metastases are based on size, with a short-axis diameter of greater than either 8 or 10 mm as a common threshold for identifying nodal disease. The morphologic techniques have a relatively low sensitivity for detecting nodal metastases in endometrial cancer, ranging from 18% to 66%.[90–94] When endometrial cancer

spreads outside the uterus, the most common patterns of spread are lymphatic to the pelvic and/or PALN, within the peritoneal cavity (most commonly with papillary serous histology), and hematogenous spread to lung, bones, or vagina. Pelvic lymph nodes are clearly the most common of the sites of metastases at the time of initial diagnosis, with most of the other sites being occult and presenting as sites of recurrence. The role of preoperative imaging is to identify patients with metastatic disease that require either more extensive surgery or a systemic therapy approach, such as chemotherapy.

The most common site of metastases at the time of diagnosis is to the regional lymph nodes; this is often micrometastatic disease for which FDG-PET/CT has a low sensitivity. In a study of 30 patients, Suzuki and colleagues[95] assessed 30 women with endometrial cancer and found that preoperative PET failed to detect the 5 cases of positive lymph node involvement when the size was 0.6 cm or less. PET was more sensitive than either CT or MR imaging for identifying other extranodal metastatic disease. The sensitivity of PET for detection of metastatic lesions was superior (83.3%) to that of CT/MR imaging (66.7%). Kitajima and colleagues[96] also investigated the accuracy of PET/CT in detecting nodal metastasis in 40 women with endometrial cancer.[95] Their study objective "was to evaluate the accuracy of integrated PET and CT (PET/CT) using ^{18}F-FDG in detecting pelvic and PALN metastasis in patients with endometrial cancer, using surgical and histopathologic findings as the reference standard." Ten of the 40 women in their study had positive lymph nodes, with this high percentage suggesting that they included a relatively high-risk population. The investigators also found a higher sensitivity for detecting lymph node metastases as the size of the involved node increased. With 60 total positive nodes found in these 10 node-positive women, the sensitivity for detecting metastatic lesions 4 mm or less in diameter was 16.7% (4/24); it was 66.7% (14/21) for lesions between 5 and 9 mm; and 93.3% (14/15) for lesions 10 mm or larger.

Because all these women require a surgical procedure unless extensive metastatic disease is present, there is no apparent benefit to the addition of preoperative staging with CT or PET scan. This finding is not surprising, given the recent cooperative group trials showing no survival benefit to systematic pelvic lymphadenectomy, which is likely more sensitive than any imaging technique. In the future, a randomized study of

PET/CT imaging as compared with surgical staging and with no extended staging in a high-risk patient population would be useful in further defining the best patient management.

Treatment

The typical treatment approach for a woman with endometrial cancer is to perform a total hysterectomy and bilateral salpingo-oophorectomy, with or without lymph node dissection. This procedure can be performed by laparotomy or by using minimally invasive surgery with laparoscopy alone or with robotic assistance. The GOG Lap 2 trial showed no significant difference in survival for women treated with laparotomy versus minimally invasive surgery. The laparoscopy arm of this study had fewer moderate and severe postoperative complications and shorter length of stay.[97] Surgical assessment of the pelvic and PALNs has been the reference standard for evaluating the extent of disease in endometrial cancer since the adoption of the 1988 version of FIGO staging. Despite the decision by FIGO to include complete surgical staging with lymph node dissection, many surgeons perform only selective lymph node dissection or removal, based on prognostic factors and intraoperative findings. The risks of lymph node dissection include the acute concerns of bleeding, prolonged operative time, increased risk of thromboembolic disease, and the delayed risk of lymphedema and lymphocyst. A recent phase 3 randomized clinical trial evaluated the survival benefits of systematic pelvic lymphadenectomy for women with intermediate or high-risk early-stage endometrial cancer, defined as FIGO (1988) stage IA or B, and high-risk histology, or FIGO Stage IC/IIA. The study took place in 85 centers in 4 different countries, and included 1408 women.[98] This ASTEC (A Study of the Treatment of Endometrial Cancer) study showed no progression-free or overall survival benefit for women who underwent complete surgical staging with systematic lymphadenectomy.[98] The 5-year overall survival was 81% in the standard surgery group and 80% in the lymphadenectomy group. Critics of the study express concern that women with surgically positive pelvic lymph nodes were still randomized to receive or not receive pelvic radiotherapy. Lymphadenectomy is considered by many to be the gold standard for assessing regional metastasis, but the fact that a randomized trial showed no survival benefit suggests otherwise. Either the sensitivity of this assessment of regional metastases is too low or the results do not affect survival because they herald distant metastatic disease.

Posttreatment Surveillance

The use of an expensive surveillance tool such as FDG-PET/CT to detect recurrent disease that is rarely cured is difficult to justify. In surgical stage I endometrial cancer, the 5-year disease-free survival exceeds 90% and therefore many repeat studies would be required to detect an unlikely recurrence. The most common site of recurrence is the vagina, which can be detected clinically but may be obscured on PET/CT by the adjacent contrast within the bladder. The use of FDG imaging for recurrence surveillance was studied by Saga and colleagues[99] in a retrospective evaluation of 21 women treated surgically for endometrial cancer. FDG imaging was found to improve "diagnostic accuracy," with a sensitivity of 100%, a specificity of 88%, and an accuracy of 93%, when compared with CT or MR imaging. In an earlier publication, Belhocine and colleagues[25] studied 34 women in posttreatment surveillance, evaluating the accurate localization of suspected recurrence and detection of occult or asymptomatic recurrence, and reported a sensitivity of 96%, specificity of 78%, and accuracy of 90%. More recently, Park and colleagues[100] reported on 88 women who underwent PET/CT as posttreatment surveillance. In this study, 66 women were asymptomatic and without evidence of disease. The investigators found that treatment was changed in 22% of patients by introducing PET or PET/CT into their posttreatment surveillance. Furthermore, they note that PET/CT is highly effective in discriminating true from suspected recurrence. These high percentages imply that Park and colleagues were monitoring a high-risk patient population in this retrospective evaluation.

The routine use of FDG imaging as posttreatment surveillance has not been studied in a randomized trial and is unlikely to be cost effective. Recurrence of endometrial cancer is relatively uncommon, and timing of the diagnosis rarely affects the likelihood of salvage. The use of PET/CT may be useful, however, in treatment planning for women found to have recurrent disease.

Recurrent Endometrial Cancer

The common sites of endometrial cancer recurrence are the vagina, pelvic and PALNs, the peritoneal cavity, and lungs. Other sites of hematogenous spread, such as bone, liver, and brain, can occur but are uncommon. Vaginal recurrence of this cancer is the most common site, occurring in approximately 7% of cases. It is detected by the occurrence of bleeding and is readily apparent on vaginal examination. Vaginal recurrence can be successfully treated in 50% to 75% of cases. Other sites of recurrence, with the exception of isolated pelvic lymph nodes, are rarely salvaged. Detection of other sites of metastases generally requires imaging with CT, MR imaging, or PET/CT. Routine surveillance imaging has not proved to be effective, and likely will not be until a curative treatment for this recurrent metastatic disease is found.

FDG imaging has been shown to play an important role in the decision-making process for women with known recurrent endometrial cancer. For women with an isolated site of recurrence, surgery and/or radiotherapy may be either curative or provide effective palliation, but with multifocal recurrent disease, only palliative chemotherapy is indicated. Kitajima and colleagues[101] studied PET versus CT performance in 90 women with recurrent endometrial or cervical cancer, and found that PET improved the sensitivity and specificity for assessing the extent of disease when compared with CT. These investigators also noted that in 42% of patients, PET results led to a change of management.

Research Concepts Using Other Tracers

Studies using ^{18}F-17β-estradiol (FES) and FDG-PET have been reported in the literature by Yoshida and colleagues.[102,103] These investigators found that FES-PET is more useful in monitoring hormone therapy, especially in endometrial hyperplasia, than FDG-PET. This differential monitoring of PET signals certainly could provide valuable insights into the management of recurrent disease or fertility-sparing interventions where hormone receptor status could inform the decision to treat a woman with progestin or antiestrogen therapy rather than chemotherapy. These treatment decision strategies, however, are only theoretical and have not yet been investigated.

Endometrial cancer is a common malignancy that usually has a good prognosis. Given the favorable outcomes generally seen, there is no apparent benefit to extensive surgical or radiologic staging of these women. The utility of FDG-PET/CT is confined to clarifying the extent and location of recurrent disease, thus assisting in the individualization of salvage therapy decisions.

SUMMARY

The experience of recent years has shown that intensive teamwork yields the best results in treating gynecologic cancer patients. The team is composed of several key participants. The imaging department uses state-of-the-art technologies and accumulated experience to reach the most accurate diagnosis. The skilled physician uses innovative tools and minimally invasive procedures to achieve impressive surgical results. The modern pathologist accurately characterizes the tumor. The oncologist aptly provides the appropriate treatment according to the type and location of the tumor, combining radiation, chemotherapy, and various biologic substances.

To overcome the limitation of traditional diagnostic modalities, a combination of anatomic and metabolic imaging has been implanted in clinical practice over the last decade. This combination enhances the clinician's ability to make critical decisions in treating difficult scenarios in various gynecologic cancer patients. Further research is needed to evaluate the efficacy of PET/CT as the diagnostic modality of choice in daily clinical practice.

REFERENCES

1. Ellenson LH, Wu TC. Focus on endometrial and cervical cancer. Cancer Cell 2004;5(6):533–8.
2. Walboomers JM, Jacobs MV, Manos MM, et al. Human papillomavirus is a necessary cause of invasive cervical cancer worldwide. J Pathol 1999;189(1):12–9.
3. Markowitz LE, Dunne EF, Saraiya M, et al. Quadrivalent human papillomavirus vaccine: recommendations of the advisory committee on immunization practices (ACIP). MMWR Recomm Rep 2007;56(RR-2):1–24.
4. Lagasse LD, Creasman WT, Shingleton HM, et al. Results and complications of operative staging in cervical cancer: experience of the Gynecologic Oncology Group. Gynecol Oncol 1980;9(1):90–8.
5. Peters WA 3rd, Liu PY, Barrett RJ 2nd, et al. Concurrent chemotherapy and pelvic radiation therapy compared with pelvic radiation therapy alone as adjuvant therapy after radical surgery in high-risk early-stage cancer of the cervix. J Clin Oncol 2000;18(8):1606–13.
6. Rose PG, Bundy BN, Watkins EB, et al. Concurrent cisplatin-based radiotherapy and chemotherapy for locally advanced cervical cancer. N Engl J Med 1999;340(15):1144–53.
7. Sedlis A, Bundy BN, Rotman MZ, et al. A randomized trial of pelvic radiation therapy versus no further therapy in selected patients with stage IB carcinoma of the cervix after radical hysterectomy and pelvic lymphadenectomy: a Gynecologic Oncology Group Study. Gynecol Oncol 1999;73(2):177–83.

8. Grigsby PW, Siegel BA, Dehdashti F. Lymph node staging by positron emission tomography in patients with carcinoma of the cervix. J Clin Oncol 2001;19(17):3745–9.

9. Burnett AF, Roman LD, O'Meara AT, et al. Radical vaginal trachelectomy and pelvic lymphadenectomy for preservation of fertility in early cervical carcinoma. Gynecol Oncol 2003;88(3):419–23.

10. Long HJ 3rd, Bundy BN, Grendys EC Jr, et al. Randomized phase III trial of cisplatin with or without topotecan in carcinoma of the uterine cervix: a Gynecologic Oncology Group Study. J Clin Oncol 2005;23(21):4626–33.

11. Whitcomb BP. Gynecologic malignancies. Surg Clin North Am 2008;88(2):301–17, vi.

12. Magne N, Chargari C, Vicenzi L, et al. New trends in the evaluation and treatment of cervix cancer: the role of FDG-PET. Cancer Treat Rev 2008;34(8):671–81.

13. Grigsby PW. The prognostic value of PET and PET/CT in cervical cancer. Cancer Imaging 2008;8:146–55.

14. Narayan K, Hicks RJ, Jobling T, et al. A comparison of MRI and PET scanning in surgically staged locoregionally advanced cervical cancer: potential impact on treatment. Int J Gynecol Cancer 2001;11(4):263–71.

15. Singh AK, Grigsby PW, Dehdashti F, et al. FDG-PET lymph node staging and survival of patients with FIGO stage IIIb cervical carcinoma. Int J Radiat Oncol Biol Phys 2003;56(2):489–93.

16. Yeh LS, Hung YC, Shen YY, et al. Detecting para-aortic lymph nodal metastasis by positron emission tomography of ^{18}F-fluorodeoxyglucose in advanced cervical cancer with negative magnetic resonance imaging findings. Oncol Rep 2002;9(6):1289–92.

17. Yen TC, Ng KK, Ma SY, et al. Value of dual-phase 2-fluoro-2-deoxy-D-glucose positron emission tomography in cervical cancer. J Clin Oncol 2003;21(19):3651–8.

18. Amit A, Beck D, Lowenstein L, et al. The role of hybrid PET/CT in the evaluation of patients with cervical cancer. Gynecol Oncol 2006;100(1):65–9.

19. Grigsby PW. PET/CT imaging to guide cervical cancer therapy. Future Oncol 2009;5(7):953–8.

20. Rose PG, Adler LP, Rodriguez M, et al. Positron emission tomography for evaluating para-aortic nodal metastasis in locally advanced cervical cancer before surgical staging: a surgicopathologic study. J Clin Oncol 1999;17(1):41–5.

21. Wright JD, Dehdashti F, Herzog TJ, et al. Preoperative lymph node staging of early-stage cervical carcinoma by [^{18}F]-fluoro-2-deoxy-D-glucose-positron emission tomography. Cancer 2005;104(11):2484–91.

22. Loft A, Berthelsen AK, Roed H, et al. The diagnostic value of PET/CT scanning in patients with cervical cancer: a prospective study. Gynecol Oncol 2007;106(1):29–34.

23. Qiu JT, Ho KC, Lai CH, et al. Supraclavicular lymph node metastases in cervical cancer. Eur J Gynaecol Oncol 2007;28(1):33–8.

24. Tsai CS, Chang TC, Lai CH, et al. Preliminary report of using FDG-PET to detect extrapelvic lesions in cervical cancer patients with enlarged pelvic lymph nodes on MRI/CT. Int J Radiat Oncol Biol Phys 2004;58(5):1506–12.

25. Belhocine T, De Barsy C, Hustinx R, et al. Usefulness of (18)F-FDG PET in the post-therapy surveillance of endometrial carcinoma. Eur J Nucl Med Mol Imaging 2002;29(9):1132–9.

26. Brooks RA, Rader JS, Dehdashti F, et al. Surveillance FDG-PET detection of asymptomatic recurrences in patients with cervical cancer. Gynecol Oncol 2009;112(1):104–9.

27. Grigsby PW, Siegel BA, Dehdashti F, et al. Post-therapy [^{18}F] fluorodeoxyglucose positron emission tomography in carcinoma of the cervix: response and outcome. J Clin Oncol 2004;22(11):2167–71.

28. Tran BN, Grigsby PW, Dehdashti F, et al. Occult supraclavicular lymph node metastasis identified by FDG-PET in patients with carcinoma of the uterine cervix. Gynecol Oncol 2003;90(3):572–6.

29. Bodurka-Bevers D, Morris M, Eifel PJ, et al. Post-therapy surveillance of women with cervical cancer: an outcomes analysis. Gynecol Oncol 2000;78(2):187–93.

30. Chien CR, Ting LL, Hsieh CY, et al. Post-radiation Pap smear for Chinese patients with cervical cancer: a ten-year follow-up. Eur J Gynaecol Oncol 2005;26(6):619–22.

31. Shield PW, Daunter B, Wright RG. Post-irradiation cytology of cervical cancer patients. Cytopathology 1992;3(3):167–82.

32. Schwarz JK, Grigsby PW, Dehdashti F, et al. The role of ^{18}F-FDG PET in assessing therapy response in cancer of the cervix and ovaries. J Nucl Med 2009;50(Suppl 1):64S–73S.

33. Morice P, Deyrolle C, Rey A, et al. Value of routine follow-up procedures for patients with stage I/II cervical cancer treated with combined surgery-radiation therapy. Ann Oncol 2004;15(2):218–23.

34. Permuth-Wey J, Sellers TA. Epidemiology of ovarian cancer. Methods Mol Biol 2009;472:413–37.

35. Auersperg N, Wong AS, Choi KC, et al. Ovarian surface epithelium: biology, endocrinology, and pathology. Endocr Rev 2001;22(2):255–88.

36. Riman T, Nilsson S, Persson IR. Review of epidemiological evidence for reproductive and hormonal factors in relation to the risk of epithelial ovarian

malignancies. Acta Obstet Gynecol Scand 2004; 83(9):783–95.

37. Edwards BK, Brown ML, Wingo PA, et al. Annual report to the nation on the status of cancer, 1975-2002, featuring population-based trends in cancer treatment. J Natl Cancer Inst 2005;97(19):1407–27.

38. Ziogas A, Gildea M, Cohen P, et al. Cancer risk estimates for family members of a population-based family registry for breast and ovarian cancer. Cancer Epidemiol Biomarkers Prev 2000; 9(1):103–11.

39. Malander S, Rambech E, Kristoffersson U, et al. The contribution of the hereditary nonpolyposis colorectal cancer syndrome to the development of ovarian cancer. Gynecol Oncol 2006;101(2): 238–43.

40. Siskind V, Green A, Bain C, et al. Beyond ovulation: oral contraceptives and epithelial ovarian cancer. Epidemiology 2000;11(2):106–10.

41. Schutter EM, Kenemans P, Sohn C, et al. Diagnostic value of pelvic examination, ultrasound, and serum CA 125 in postmenopausal women with a pelvic mass. An international multicenter study. Cancer 1994;74(4):1398–406.

42. Schutter EM, Sohn C, Kristen P, et al. Estimation of probability of malignancy using a logistic model combining physical examination, ultrasound, serum CA 125, and serum CA 72-4 in postmenopausal women with a pelvic mass: an international multicenter study. Gynecol Oncol 1998;69(1): 56–63.

43. Burghardt E, Lahousen M, Stettner H. The significance of pelvic and para-aortic lymphadenectomy in the operative treatment of ovarian cancer. Baillieres Clin Obstet Gynaecol 1989;3(1):157–65.

44. Burghardt E, Pickel H, Lahousen M, et al. Pelvic lymphadenectomy in operative treatment of ovarian cancer. Am J Obstet Gynecol 1986; 155(2):315–9.

45. Dauplat J, Hacker NF, Nieberg RK, et al. Distant metastases in epithelial ovarian carcinoma. Cancer 1987;60(7):1561–6.

46. Julian CG, Goss J, Blanchard K, et al. Biologic behavior of primary ovarian malignancy. Obstet Gynecol 1974;44(6):873–84.

47. Brooks SE. Preoperative evaluation of patients with suspected ovarian cancer. Gynecol Oncol 1994;55 (3 Pt 2):S80–90.

48. Curtin JP. Management of the adnexal mass. Gynecol Oncol 1994;55(3 Pt 2):S42–6.

49. Ind TE, Granowska M, Britton KE, et al. Peroperative radioimmunodetection of ovarian carcinoma using a hand-held gamma detection probe. Br J Cancer 1994;70(6):1263–6.

50. Kinkel K, Hricak H, Lu Y, et al. US characterization of ovarian masses: a meta-analysis. Radiology 2000;217(3):803–11.

51. Hewitt MJ, Anderson K, Hall GD, et al. Women with peritoneal carcinomatosis of unknown origin: Efficacy of image-guided biopsy to determine site-specific diagnosis. BJOG 2007;114(1):46–50.

52. Goff BA, Matthews BJ, Larson EH, et al. Predictors of comprehensive surgical treatment in patients with ovarian cancer. Cancer 2007;109(10): 2031–42.

53. Le T, Adolph A, Krepart GV, et al. The benefits of comprehensive surgical staging in the management of early-stage epithelial ovarian carcinoma. Gynecol Oncol 2002;85(2):351–5.

54. Eisenkop SM. Commenting on centralizing surgery for gynecologic oncology: a strategy assuring better quality treatment? (89:4-8) by Karsten Munstedt, et al. Gynecol Oncol 2004;94(2):605–6 [author reply: 606–7].

55. Munstedt K, von Georgi R, Misselwitz B, et al. Centralizing surgery for gynecologic oncology—a strategy assuring better quality treatment? Gynecol Oncol 2003;89(1):4–8.

56. Boente MP, Chi DS, Hoskins WJ. The role of surgery in the management of ovarian cancer: primary and interval cytoreductive surgery. Semin Oncol 1998;25(3):326–34.

57. Chi DS, Eisenhauer EL, Lang J, et al. What is the optimal goal of primary cytoreductive surgery for bulky stage IIIC epithelial ovarian carcinoma (EOC)? Gynecol Oncol 2006;103(2):559–64.

58. Eisenkop SM, Spirtos NM, Lin WC. "Optimal" cytoreduction for advanced epithelial ovarian cancer: a commentary. Gynecol Oncol 2006;103(1): 329–35.

59. Winter WE 3rd, Maxwell GL, Tian C, et al. Tumor residual after surgical cytoreduction in prediction of clinical outcome in stage IV epithelial ovarian cancer: a Gynecologic Oncology Group study. J Clin Oncol 2008;26(1):83–9.

60. Eisenhauer EL, Abu-Rustum NR, Sonoda Y, et al. The effect of maximal surgical cytoreduction on sensitivity to platinum-taxane chemotherapy and subsequent survival in patients with advanced ovarian cancer. Gynecol Oncol 2008;108(2): 276–81.

61. Redman CW, Warwick J, Luesley DM, et al. Intervention debulking surgery in advanced epithelial ovarian cancer. Br J Obstet Gynaecol 1994;101 (2):142–6.

62. Aletti GD, Gostout BS, Podratz KC, et al. Ovarian cancer surgical resectability: relative impact of disease, patient status, and surgeon. Gynecol Oncol 2006;100(1):33–7.

63. van der Burg ME, van Lent M, Buyse M, et al. The effect of debulking surgery after induction chemotherapy on the prognosis in advanced epithelial ovarian cancer. Gynecological Cancer Cooperative Group of the European Organization for Research

and Treatment of Cancer. N Engl J Med 1995;332: 629–34.

64. Rose PG, Nerenstone S, Brady MF, et al. Secondary surgical cytoreduction for advanced ovarian carcinoma. N Engl J Med 2004;351(24): 2489–97.

65. Wenzel L, Huang HQ, Monk BJ, et al. Quality-of-life comparisons in a randomized trial of interval secondary cytoreduction in advanced ovarian carcinoma: a Gynecologic Oncology Group study. J Clin Oncol 2005;23(24):5605–12.

66. Ozols RF, Bundy BN, Greer BE, et al. Phase III trial of carboplatin and paclitaxel compared with cisplatin and paclitaxel in patients with optimally resected stage III ovarian cancer: a Gynecologic Oncology Group study. J Clin Oncol 2003;21(17): 3194–200.

67. Greimel ER, Bjelic-Radisic V, Pfisterer J, et al. Randomized study of the Arbeitsgemeinschaft Gynaekologische Onkologie Ovarian Cancer Study Group comparing quality of life in patients with ovarian cancer treated with cisplatin/paclitaxel versus carboplatin/paclitaxel. J Clin Oncol 2006; 24(4):579–86.

68. Einzig AI, Wiernik PH, Sasloff J, et al. Phase II study and long-term follow-up of patients treated with taxol for advanced ovarian adenocarcinoma. J Clin Oncol 1992;10(11):1748–53.

69. Heintz AP, Odicino F, Maisonneuve P, et al. Carcinoma of the ovary. FIGO 6th annual report on the results of treatment in gynecological cancer. Int J Gynaecol Obstet 2006;95(Suppl 1):S161–92.

70. Berek JS, Trope C, Vergote I. Surgery during chemotherapy and at relapse of ovarian cancer. Ann Oncol 1999;10(Suppl 1):3–7.

71. McGuire WP, Hoskins WJ, Brady MF, et al. Cyclophosphamide and cisplatin compared with paclitaxel and cisplatin in patients with stage III and stage IV ovarian cancer. N Engl J Med 1996; 334(1):1–6.

72. Risum S, Hogdall C, Loft A, et al. Does the use of diagnostic PET/CT cause stage migration in patients with primary advanced ovarian cancer? Gynecol Oncol 2010;116(3):395–8.

73. Risum S, Hogdall C, Loft A, et al. The diagnostic value of PET/CT for primary ovarian cancer—a prospective study. Gynecol Oncol 2007;105(1):145–9.

74. Gu P, Pan LL, Wu SQ, et al. CA 125, PET alone, PET-CT, CT and MRI in diagnosing recurrent ovarian carcinoma: a systematic review and meta-analysis. Eur J Radiol 2009;71(1):164–74.

75. Moore RG, MacLaughlan S, Bast RC Jr. Current state of biomarker development for clinical application in epithelial ovarian cancer. Gynecol Oncol 2010;116(2):240–5.

76. Agress H Jr, Cooper BZ. Detection of clinically unexpected malignant and premalignant tumors

with whole-body FDG PET: histopathologic comparison. Radiology 2004;230(2):417–22.

77. Milam RA, Milam MR, Iyer RB. Detection of early-stage ovarian cancer by FDG-PET-CT in a patient with BRCA2-positive breast cancer. J Clin Oncol 2007;25(35):5657–8.

78. Barnholtz-Sloan JS, Schwartz AG, Qureshi F, et al. Ovarian cancer: changes in patterns at diagnosis and relative survival over the last three decades. Am J Obstet Gynecol 2003;189(4):1120–7.

79. Tailor A, Bourne TH, Campbell S, et al. Results from an ultrasound-based familial ovarian cancer screening clinic: a 10-year observational study. Ultrasound Obstet Gynecol 2003;21(4):378–85.

80. Karlan BY, Baldwin RL, Lopez-Luevanos E, et al. Peritoneal serous papillary carcinoma, a phenotypic variant of familial ovarian cancer: implications for ovarian cancer screening. Am J Obstet Gynecol 1999;180(4):917–28.

81. Olivier RI, Lubsen-Brandsma MA, Verhoef S, et al. CA125 and transvaginal ultrasound monitoring in high-risk women cannot prevent the diagnosis of advanced ovarian cancer. Gynecol Oncol 2006; 100(1):20–6.

82. Gadducci A, Cosio S. Surveillance of patients after initial treatment of ovarian cancer. Crit Rev Oncol Hematol 2009;71(1):43–52.

83. Jung DC, Kang S, Kim MJ, et al. Multidetector CT predictors of incomplete resection in primary cytoreduction of patients with advanced ovarian cancer. Eur Radiol 2010;20(1):100–7.

84. Gadducci A, Cosio S, Zola P, et al. Surveillance procedures for patients treated for epithelial ovarian cancer: a review of the literature. Int J Gynecol Cancer 2007;17(1):21–31.

85. Parkin DM, Bray F, Ferlay J, et al. Global cancer statistics, 2002. CA Cancer J Clin 2005;55(2): 74–108.

86. Schink JC, Rademaker AW, Miller DS, et al. Tumor size in endometrial cancer. Cancer 1991;67(11): 2791–4.

87. Karlsson B, Granberg S, Wikland M, et al. Transvaginal ultrasonography of the endometrium in women with postmenopausal bleeding—a Nordic multicenter study. Am J Obstet Gynecol 1995; 172(5):1488–94.

88. Gupta JK, Chien PF, Voit D, et al. Ultrasonographic endometrial thickness for diagnosing endometrial pathology in women with postmenopausal bleeding: a meta-analysis. Acta Obstet Gynecol Scand 2002;81(9):799–816.

89. Tabor A, Watt HC, Wald NJ. Endometrial thickness as a test for endometrial cancer in women with postmenopausal vaginal bleeding. Obstet Gynecol 2002;99(4):663–70.

90. Hricak H, Rubinstein LV, Gherman GM, et al. MR imaging evaluation of endometrial carcinoma

results of an NCI cooperative study. Radiology 1991;179(3):829–32.

91. Connor JP, Andrews JI, Anderson B, et al. Computed tomography in endometrial carcinoma. Obstet Gynecol 2000;95(5):692–6.

92. Manfredi R, Mirk P, Maresca G, et al. Local-regional staging of endometrial carcinoma: role of MR imaging in surgical planning. Radiology 2004;231(2):372–8.

93. Rockall AG, Sohaib SA, Harisinghani MG, et al. Diagnostic performance of nanoparticle-enhanced magnetic resonance imaging in the diagnosis of lymph node metastases in patients with endometrial and cervical cancer. J Clin Oncol 2005;23(12):2813–21.

94. Sugiyama T, Nishida T, Ushijima K, et al. Detection of lymph node metastasis in ovarian carcinoma and uterine corpus carcinoma by preoperative computerized tomography or magnetic resonance imaging. J Obstet Gynaecol (Tokyo 1995) 1995; 21(6):551–6.

95. Suzuki R, Miyagi E, Takahashi N, et al. Validity of positron emission tomography using fluoro-2-deoxyglucose for the preoperative evaluation of endometrial cancer. Int J Gynecol Cancer 2007; 17(4):890–6.

96. Kitajima K, Murakami K, Yamasaki E, et al. Accuracy of ^{18}F-FDG PET/CT in detecting pelvic and paraaortic lymph node metastasis in patients with endometrial cancer. Am J Roentgenol 2008; 190(6):1652–8.

97. Walker JL, Piedmonte MR, Spirtos NM, et al. Laparoscopy compared with laparotomy for comprehensive surgical staging of uterine cancer: Gynecologic Oncology Group Study LAP2. J Clin Oncol 2009;27(32):5331–6.

98. ASTEC study group, Kitchener H, Swart AM, et al. Efficacy of systematic pelvic lymphadenectomy in endometrial cancer (MRC ASTEC trial): a randomised study. Lancet 2009; 373(9658):125–36.

99. Saga T, Higashi T, Ishimori T, et al. Clinical value of FDG-PET in the follow up of post-operative patients with endometrial cancer. Ann Nucl Med 2003;17(3): 197–203.

100. Park JY, Kim EN, Kim DY, et al. Clinical impact of positron emission tomography or positron emission tomography/computed tomography in the post-therapy surveillance of endometrial carcinoma: evaluation of 88 patients. Int J Gynecol Cancer 2008;18(6):1332–8.

101. Kitajima K, Murakami K, Yamasaki E, et al. Performance of integrated FDG-PET/contrast-enhanced CT in the diagnosis of recurrent uterine cancer: comparison with PET and enhanced CT. Eur J Nucl Med Mol Imaging 2009;36(3):362–72.

102. Yoshida Y, Kurokawa T, Sawamura Y, et al. The positron emission tomography with F18 17beta-estradiol has the potential to benefit diagnosis and treatment of endometrial cancer. Gynecol Oncol 2007;104(3):764–6.

103. Pecorelli S. Revised FIGO staging for carcinoma of the vulva, cervix, and endometrium. Int J Gynaecol Obstet 2009;105(2):103–4.

Radiological Assessment of Gynecologic Malignancies

Daniel J. Bell, MBChB*, Harpreet K. Pannu, MD

KEYWORDS

- Gynecology • Computed tomography
- Magnetic resonance imaging • Ultrasonography
- Sonography • Malignancy

Patients with gynecologic malignancies are evaluated with a combination of clinical and diagnostic imaging methods. Imaging with ultrasonography (US), computed tomography (CT), and magnetic resonance (MR) has a role in detection of and characterizing gynecologic masses, and can supplement clinical staging, help in preoperative planning for surgery, and assess patients for tumor recurrence. US has a primary role in detecting and characterizing endometrial and adnexal pathology. The role of CT is primarily to stage malignancy and detect recurrence, although it can also detect larger gynecologic masses. MR imaging has added specificity over US for lesion characterization, superior contrast resolution for visualizing uterine and adnexal masses, and is also useful for staging gynecologic malignancies. This review focuses on the radiologic imaging of the 3 most common gynecologic tumors: endometrial, cervical, and ovarian carcinomas.

ENDOMETRIAL CARCINOMA

Endometrial carcinoma is the most common gynecologic malignancy, with approximately 40,000 new cases diagnosed in the United States each year.[1] Pathologically and clinically, endometrial cancer is divided into 2 main subtypes: endometrioid (Type I) and nonendometrioid (Type II) tumors. Endometrioid histology is seen in 80% to 90% of patients.[2] Patients are usually perimenopausal

and have risk factors associated with increased estrogen exposure such as nulliparity, chronic anovulation, and obesity. The tumors are confined, as a rule, to the uterus and have a good prognosis. On the other hand, nonendometrioid subtypes are seen in older multiparous women, usually without increased estrogen exposure.[3] The most common forms are uterine papillary serous carcinoma and clear cell carcinoma. These tumors have a high propensity for myometrial and vascular invasion as well as peritoneal carcinomatosis, and carry a poorer prognosis than endometrioid carcinoma.[4] Painless bleeding is the most frequent presenting symptom of endometrial cancer. Effective steps for the evaluation of patients' postmenopausal bleeding (PMB) are transvaginal sonography (TVS), endometrial biopsy (EMB), and hysteroscopy.[5] Once malignancy is detected, tumor bulk as well as local and distant spread can be assessed with imaging before surgical staging.

Role of Imaging in Primary Tumor Assessment

The role of imaging is twofold: to evaluate the symptomatic patient for a possible endometrial abnormality, and to characterize and stage disease in those with known pathology. Initial evaluation uses US to assess endometrial thickness and appearance. The normal endometrium is homogeneously hyperechoic and thin, but is thickened and heterogeneous with hyperplasia, polyps,

Department of Radiology, Memorial Sloan-Kettering Cancer Center, 1275 York Avenue, New York City, NY 10065, USA
* Corresponding author.
E-mail address: belld@mskcc.org

PET Clin 5 (2010) 407–423
doi:10.1016/j.cpet.2010.07.002
1556-8598/10/$ — see front matter © 2010 Elsevier Inc. All rights reserved.

pet.theclinics.com

and cancer (**Fig. 1**). The consensus statement from the Society of Radiologists in Ultrasound has defined an endometrial thickness of 5 mm or greater on TVS as being abnormal in patients with painless PMB.[5] Using a threshold of 5 mm, the sensitivity of TVS approaches that of endometrial biopsy, and had a sensitivity of 96% for detecting an endometrial abnormality in patients with cancer in a meta-analysis of 35 studies.[6]

The negative predictive value (NPV) of TVS is high and can be used to obviate biopsy. However, the specificity is decreased in patients who are on hormone replacement therapy or medications such as tamoxifen. Also, endometrial thickening due to hyperplasia, polyps, fibroids, and malignancy can be difficult to distinguish on routine TVS. Presence of an echogenic lesion with a vascular stalk favors a polyp while fibroids are hypoechoic or heterogeneous and broad-based.

In equivocal cases, sonohysterography can be performed to better assess the endometrium. With this technique, the endometrial cavity is distended with saline through a small-bore catheter tip placed in the cervix while real-time TVS images of the lining are acquired to assess for smooth versus irregular thickening and masses. The endoluminal distention achieved aids in both the detection and characterization of endometrial masses. In a study of 114 patients who had an abnormal sonohysterogram, 14% had a normal-appearing endometrium on routine TVS while the sonohysterogram showed polyps and/or submucosal fibroids (**Fig. 2**).[7] Sonohysterography detected the etiology of PMB in 70% of 98 patients for an

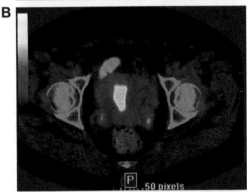

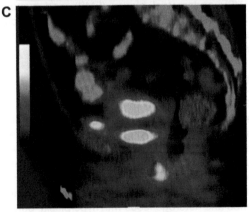

Fig. 1. Endometrioid-type endometrial carcinoma in a 70-year-old woman with breast carcinoma following an incidental finding of an ^{18}F-fluorodeoxyglucose (FDG)-avid endometrium on PET/CT performed at staging. (*A*) Longitudinal transvaginal sonogram of the uterus shows the diffusely thickened endometrium. PET/CT (*B*) axial and (*C*) sagittal images show an FDG-avid focus in the endometrium.

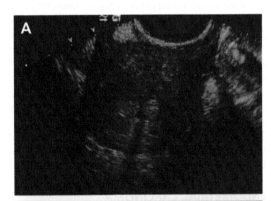

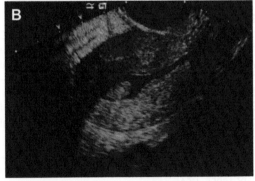

Fig. 2. Endometrial polyps in a 40-year-old woman with breast carcinoma. (*A*) Transverse and (*B*) longitudinal sonohysterogram demonstrates the presence of 2 echogenic endometrial polyps.

overall sensitivity of 98%, specificity of 88%, positive predictive value (PPV) of 94%, and NPV of 97%.[8] The appearance of endometrial cancer is variable, but includes thickening and a polypoid mass.[9] Using the criteria of a focal heterogeneous mass projecting into the endometrial cavity or focal thickening greater than 4 mm, a study of 88 women undergoing sonohysterography detected endometrial cancer in 8 of 9 women positive for malignancy at surgery for a sensitivity of 89%, specificity of 46%, PPV of 16%, and NPV of 97%.[10]

Once endometrial malignancy is detected, preliminary staging can be done with imaging before definitive surgical staging, which remains the standard of care for endometrial carcinoma unless the patient is a poor surgical candidate. Surgical staging involves hysterectomy, bilateral salpingo-oophorectomy, peritoneal washing, and lymphadenectomy. The key factors are the histopathologic grade of the tumor and degree of myometrial involvement. Adverse features are higher tumor grade and deep myometrial invasion, as these are associated with higher stage disease such as nodal metastases.

Of the imaging modalities available, MR imaging has excellent contrast resolution and allows assessment of the entire pelvis in multiple planes without the use of ionizing radiation. The role of MR imaging is primarily to stage endometrial cancer. In unusual cases it can be also a supplemental technique to evaluate the endometrium if US or hysteroscopy cannot be performed or are equivocal. The T2-weighted and contrast-enhanced sequences are the most useful for distinguishing normal endometrium and myometrium from disease. Imaging parallel and perpendicular to the plane of the uterus optimizes visualization of the endometrial-myometrial interface. The normal endometrium is hyperintense on T2-weighted images while tumors tend to be intermediate and heterogeneous in signal intensity (**Fig. 3**).[11] Hemorrhage in the endometrial cavity can also have low signal intensity on T2 but is hyperintense on precontrast T1-weighted images. Compared with tumors, the inner myometrium or junctional zone is hypointense on T2-weighted images. The junctional zone is more conspicuous in premenopausal women but is not well seen in older postmenopausal women. Because of this limiting factor, contrast-enhanced scans have been found to be more useful because after injection of contrast the tumor enhances less than the normal myometrium and is relatively hypointense.[12,13] Invasive disease appears as a hypointense tumor

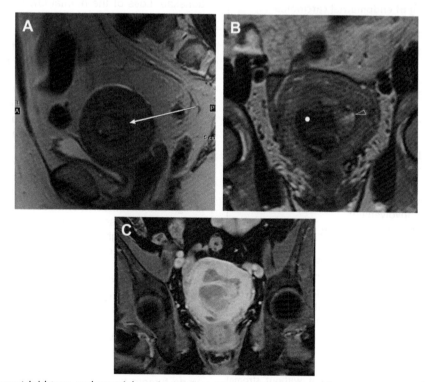

Fig. 3. Endometrioid-type endometrial carcinoma in a 60-year-old woman with postmenopausal bleeding. (*A*) Sagittal T2-weighted, (*B*) coronal T2-weighted, and (*C*) coronal T1-weighted fat-saturation post-gadolinium MR imaging show an enhancing polypoid endometrial mass in the left side of the fundus (*arrow* in *A, arrowhead* in *B*) without deep myometrial invasion. Adjacent fibroid (*white circle*) is also noted.

extending into the myometrium, with irregularity and disruption of the enhancing inner myometrium at the endometrial-myometrial interface.

The staging system for endometrial carcinoma was revised by the International Federation of Gynecology and Obstetrics (FIGO) in 2008 (**Table 1**). Tumors confined to the endometrium or having less than 50% depth of myometrial invasion are defined as Stage IA while those with 50% or more myometrial invasion are Stage IB.[14] MR imaging can assess the degree of myometrial involvement and distinguish superficial from deep invasion with a relatively high accuracy of 83% to 89%.[15–17] In a study of 101 patients, including 48 with pathologic evidence of deep myometrial invasion, 90% of patients were correctly staged by MR imaging and 10% were understaged.[18] Assessment of invasion can be difficult in the presence of coexisting benign myometrial abnormalities such as adenomyosis, as well as in patients with an indistinct junctional zone, if there is poor contrast between the tumor and normal myometrium or if tumor involves the uterine cornua.[12,19] Adenomyosis appears as heterogeneous ill-defined regions with thickening of the junctional zone and small cystic foci on T2-weighted images. The addition of dynamic contrast-enhanced images to T2-weighted images increased the accuracy for depth of myometrial invasion from 78% to 92% in a study on 50 patients.[19,20] The likelihood ratios (LR) for predicting deep myometrial invasion with contrast-enhanced MR imaging were positive LR of 10.11 and negative LR of 0.1 in a meta-analysis of 9 articles with a total of 742 patients.[21]

In addition to the myometrium, cervical stromal invasion is also evaluated on MR imaging, as it is an indication for radical hysterectomy.[4] The normal cervical stroma is hypointense on T2-weighted images and is replaced by intermediate signal intensity tumor in cases of invasion. Endocervical extension manifests as widening of the cervical canal by an inferiorly extending endometrial mass. Addition of intravenous contrast can improve detection of cervical invasion. One study has reported that MR imaging had 80% sensitivity, 96% specificity, 89% PPV, and 93% NPV for assessing cervical infiltration.[15] The new FIGO classification places endocervical glandular tumor extension into Stage I and cervical stromal invasion into Stage II.[14] With local extension of tumor beyond the uterus, there is abnormal intermediate T2 signal intensity tissue in the parametrial fat or adnexae. Loss of the normal low signal intensity wall on T2-weighted images suggests bladder or rectal invasion.[4]

Recently, there has been interest in applying diffusion-weighted imaging (DWI) to evaluate gynecologic malignancies including endometrial cancer. DWI is a noncontrast technique that assesses the random motion of water molecules in tissue. The resultant information can be qualitatively assessed or quantified by calculating the apparent diffusion coefficient (ADC) value. The "b" value or factor determines the strength of the diffusion weighting on the image. In tissues with mobile molecules such as vessels, the ADC value is high and the diffusion or motion of water results in a visual decrease in signal intensity. Conversely, in tissues with high cellularity such as tumors, the movement of water is restricted resulting in a low ADC value and high visual signal intensity. Endometrial cancer shows restricted diffusion appearing hyperintense on high b value (b = 1000 s/mm^2) images.[22,23] Combining DWI with T2-weighted images may aid in the detection of tumors.[24] The ADC values of tumor are reported to be lower than benign endometrial pathology or the normal endometrium.[22,23,25] A trend for higher grade tumors to demonstrate lower ADC values compared with those of lower grade ones has been described as well.[23,25] DWI can help supplement the contrast-enhanced scan for myometrial

Table 1
FIGO staging of endometrial carcinoma

I	Tumor confined to corpus uteri
IA	Tumor limited to endometrium or invades less than one-half of the myometrium
IB	Tumor invades one-half or more of the myometrium
II	Tumor invades cervical stroma but does not extend beyond uterus[a]
III	Local and/or regional tumor spread
IIIA	Tumor invades serosa of corpus uteri and/or adnexae
IIIB	Vaginal and/or parametrial involvement
IIIC	Metastases to pelvic and/or para-aortic nodes
IIIC1	Positive pelvic nodes
IIIC2	Positive para-aortic nodes
IV	Tumor invades bladder and/or bowel mucosa and/or distant metastases
IVA	Tumor invades bladder and/or bowel mucosa
IVB	Distant metastases

[a] Endocervical glandular involvement without stromal invasion is considered as Stage I.

From Pecorelli S. Revised FIGO staging for carcinoma of the vulva, cervix, and endometrium. Int J Gynaecol Obstet 2009;105:103–4.

invasion. In a study of 62 patients with endometrial cancer, Rechichi and colleagues[26] reported a sensitivity of 84.6% and specificity of 70.6% for DWI for depicting myometrial invasion. However, a lower accuracy of DWI compared with contrast-enhanced MR imaging has also been reported because of lower spatial resolution of DWI.[22,25] Other limitations of DWI include image degradation due to magnetic field inhomogeneity and motion artifacts and poor background signal on high b-value images. Fusion of DWI with T2-weighted images aids in anatomic localization. Normal endometrium can also have restricted diffusion, and the cutoff ADC values for distinguishing normal from cancerous tissue are not established at present.[23]

MR imaging has superior soft tissue contrast and therefore is the main imaging modality for staging endometrial cancer, with TVS and CT as alternatives if MR imaging is not available. A meta-analysis of 6 CT, 16 US, and 25 MR imaging studies showed superiority of contrast-enhanced MR imaging for myometrial invasion.[27] Endometrial/myometrial echogenicity and vascularity as well as regularity of the endometrial-myometrial interface are assessed on US.[28] Newer techniques such as contrast-enhanced and 3-dimensional US may prove helpful for endometrial cancer.[29] In a study of 35 patients with endometrial cancer, tumor conspicuity increased following injection of contrast, and a feeding vessel was seen in 77% of patients.[30] Time-intensity curves of tumor enhancement can be also generated. CT provides a rapid assessment and global overview of the abdomen and pelvis for distant metastases, and is usually readily available. Soft tissue contrast resolution of CT is lower than that of MR imaging but spatial resolution tends to be higher. Evaluation of myometrial invasion was initially hampered by imaging limited to the axial plane, while the lie of the uterus was variable and usually not perpendicular to the axial plane.[31] Current multidetector-row CT (MDCT) scanners have made thin slices, isotropic datasets, and reconstruction in multiple user-defined planes possible. Using multiplanar reconstructions and imaging 70 seconds after contrast injection on a 16-row MDCT scanner, the depth of myometrial invasion was correctly assessed in 18 of 21 patients with endometrial cancer.[32]

Role of Imaging for Assessment of Nodal and Distant Metastases, and Recurrence

Nodal metastases from endometrial cancer involve pelvic and para-aortic nodes. Tumors from the middle and inferior uterus drain to the parametrial and obturator nodes whereas those from the proximal body and fundus drain to the common iliac and para-aortic nodes.[12] Lymphatic drainage from the uterus also occurs to obturator nodes, and tumor can spread via the round ligament to inguinal nodes as well. The likelihood of nodal spread increases in the presence of greater than 50% invasion of the myometrium compared with those with lesser amount of invasion.[19] In addition to depth of myometrial invasion, the incidence of nodal disease is also linked to the tumor histologic grade. For patients with greater than 50% myometrial extension, nodal metastases occurred in 28% of those with grade 3 tumors in a series of 349 patients undergoing pelvic lymphadenectomy.[33] Lymphadenectomy is associated with morbidity, and therefore a combination of preoperative imaging and intraoperative evaluation is helpful in determining if this surgical procedure is indeed necessary in each patient.[19,34] Imaging findings suggestive of nodal involvement include a short-axis diameter greater than 1 cm and presence of necrosis.[4] However, size criteria have a wide range of sensitivities, and the addition of other techniques such as lymph node contrast agents or DWI may be helpful.[35,36] Recurrent disease occurs at the vagina, abdominal and pelvic nodes, peritoneum, and lung. MR imaging can evaluate for local disease while CT is used for surveillance.

CERVICAL CARCINOMA

Cervical carcinoma is the third most common gynecologic cancer, with an estimated 11,000 cases of invasive cancer in the United States in 2009. Incidence and mortality rates have declined over the past several decades because of screening and detection of preinvasive cervical lesions.[1] Approximately 85% of cases are squamous cell carcinoma and most of the remainder are adenocarcinoma. Uncommon subtypes include adenosquamous carcinoma, lymphoma, adenoma malignum, and small cell carcinoma, the latter tending to be locally invasive as well to have distant metastases.

Role of Imaging in Primary Tumor Assessment

Unlike endometrial cancer, the recommended staging of cervical carcinoma is clinical by physical examination, colposcopy, examination under anesthesia, non–cross-sectional imaging studies such as chest radiography, barium enema, and intravenous urography, and by endoscopic studies such as cystoscopy and rectosigmoidoscopy (Table 2). Patients are triaged to surgical or nonsurgical management based on initial

Table 2
FIGO staging of cervical carcinoma

I	Cervical carcinoma confined to cervix (extension to corpus disregarded)
IA	Invasive carcinoma diagnosed only by microscopy
IA1	Measured stromal invasion 3.0 mm or less in depth and 7.0 mm or less in horizontal spread
IA2	Measured stromal invasion more than 3.0 mm but less than 5.0 mm in depth with a horizontal spread 7.0 mm or less
IB	Clinically visible lesion confined to the cervix or preclinical lesion greater than Stage IA[a]
IB1	Clinically visible lesion 4.0 cm or less in greatest dimension
IB2	Clinically visible lesion more than 4.0 cm in greatest dimension
II	Cervical carcinoma invades beyond uterus but not to pelvic wall or to lower third of vagina
IIA	Tumor without parametrial invasion
IIA1	Clinically visible lesion 4.0 cm or less in greatest dimension
IIA2	Clinically visible lesion more than 4.0 cm in greatest dimension
IIB	Tumor with obvious parametrial invasion
III	Tumor extends to pelvic wall and/or involves lower third of vagina, and/or causes hydronephrosis or nonfunctioning kidney
IIIA	Tumor involves lower third of vagina, no extension to pelvic wall
IIIB	Tumor extends to pelvic wall and/or causes hydronephrosis or nonfunctioning kidney
IV	Cancer extends beyond true pelvis or biopsy proof of invasion of the bladder or rectal mucosa
IVA	Tumor spread to adjacent organs
IVB	Distant metastases

[a] All macroscopically visible lesions, even with superficial invasion, are Stage IB.

From Pecorelli S. Revised FIGO staging for carcinoma of the vulva, cervix, and endometrium. Int J Gynaecol Obstet 2009;105:103–4.

staging results. Clinical staging can under- or overstage patients because nodal status is not determined and parametrial assessment is limited.[37] Physical examination is also subject to interobserver variability, and discrepancies between clinical staging and surgery range from

25% in early-stage to 65% in advanced-stage disease.[38] Therefore, there has been interest in assessing the additional value of cross-sectional imaging for parametrial invasion, metastatic pelvic nodes, distant metastases, and overall improved staging of cervical cancer. If MR imaging, CT, and PET/CT are available, they can be incorporated into patient staging.

Lesion size, extension into the uterine corpus, depth of stromal invasion, parametrial spread, and pelvic adenopathy are evaluated on imaging. The primary tumor, uterine anatomy, and cervical anatomy are better seen on MR imaging due to high soft tissue contrast, whereas nodes and distant metastases are seen on both CT and MR imaging. Including images perpendicular to the endocervical canal provides a cross section of the cervix and aids in diagnosing parametrial extension. The critical distinction is between stages I and IIA, which are treated surgically, and advanced disease, stage IIB and higher, which is treated with radiation or combined chemoradiation.

On MR imaging, the primary tumor is intermediate in signal intensity on T2-weighted images and is hyperintense relative to the hypointense normal cervical stroma. Tumors can be exophytic, infiltrating, or endocervical with a barrel shape. Endovaginal and multiphase imaging following intravenous contrast may aid in the visualization of small tumors.[39,40] The margins of the tumor relative to the lower uterine segment myometrium, internal and external cervical os, and vaginal fornices are determined. Next, the integrity of the cervical stroma is assessed. An intact ring of hypointense tissue on T2-weighted images has a high NPV for parametrial invasion (**Fig. 4**). Disruption of the stromal ring, contour irregularity, and vessel abutment are suspicious for parametrial disease (**Fig. 5**) which, however, can be difficult to assess in the presence of bulky masses and full-thickness invasion of the cervical stroma. Gross parametrial mass and ureteral encasement are definitive for tumor extension (**Fig. 6**).

On CT small primary tumors are typically isodense to the cervix whereas large ones can be hypodense, heterogeneous, and necrotic. Gross parametrial spread and ureteral obstruction are similar as for MR imaging. Tumors within 3 mm of the pelvic side wall, encasement of the iliac vessels, and muscle enlargement indicate pelvic side-wall invasion. Preservation of the normal fat plane between the bladder and rectum excludes involvement while tumor abutment or abnormal wall signal intensity are suspicious for disease.

Numerous studies have evaluated the utility of MR imaging and CT for staging the local extent of cervical cancer, with variable results. A

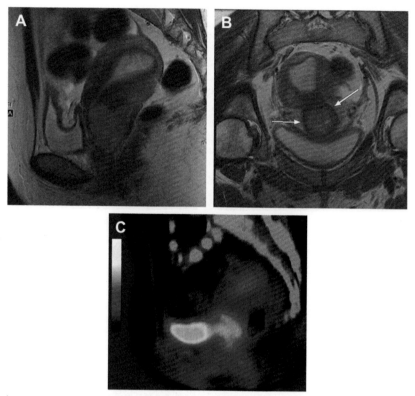

Fig. 4. Cervical carcinoma in a 40-year-old woman. (*A*) Sagittal T2-weighted MR imaging shows a bulky tumor extending from the external to internal os. (*B*) Coronal T2-weighted image demonstrates thinning of the low signal intensity cervical stroma (*arrows*) but no gross disruption to suggest parametrial invasion. (*C*) Sagittal PET/CT image shows FDG avidity of the cervical lesion.

retrospective review of the medical records of 255 patients imaged between 1992 and 2003 found clinical pelvic examination to be superior to MR imaging and CT, and had a higher sensitivity and specificity for parametrial disease.[41] However, over recent years these imaging modalities have evolved technologically and other investigators have reported relatively high accuracy for staging with MR imaging.[37,42,43] A recent study evaluating the depth of stromal invasion with MR imaging in 53 patients with stage I or IIA disease found an agreement of 75% between MR imaging and pathology for tumor infiltration of greater or less than 50% of the width of the cervical stroma.[44] The NPV of MR imaging for parametrial invasion is high. In a study on 113 patients comparing MR imaging and surgery, the NPV was 95% and the PPV 67%.[42] Microscopic disease can cause false-negative results while parametrial inflammation and stranding can lead to a false-positive diagnosis. A high sensitivity of 80% and specificity of 91% for parametrial invasion has been found with MR imaging using an endovaginal imaging coil.[40] Sensitivities and specificities of 67% to

87% and 79% to 92% have been reported for involvement of the vaginal fornices when compared with surgery.[42,44] A meta-analysis of 57 MR imaging and/or CT articles published between 1985 and 2002 found a higher sensitivity for MR imaging than with CT for parametrial invasion (74% vs 55%), with equivalent specificities.[38] MR imaging also had a higher sensitivity and specificity for bladder invasion. The utility of CT and MR imaging has been assessed in a series of articles by the American College of Radiology Imaging Network (ACRIN) and Gynecologic Oncology Group (GOG).[45–48] A multicenter study by both groups compared MR imaging, CT, and clinical staging in patients with early-stage cervical cancer imaged between 2000 and 2002, and found a lower sensitivity and specificity for disease extent compared with results from single-institution studies. MR imaging had the highest agreement with pathology for tumor size and involvement of the uterine corpus.[46] Detection of parametrial invasion and reader agreement was also higher for MR imaging than for CT.[48] For detecting malignancies of stage IIB or higher, both MR imaging

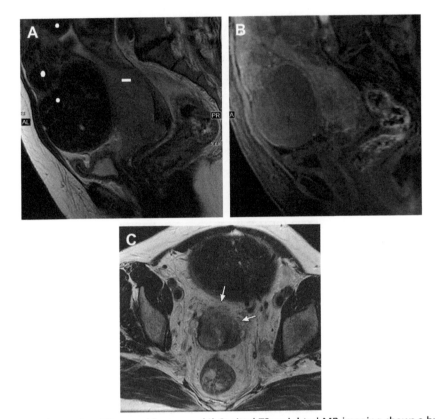

Fig. 5. Cervical carcinoma in a 50-year-old woman. (*A*) Sagittal T2-weighted MR imaging shows a bulky cervical mass (*white rectangle*) of intermediate T2 signal intensity compared with the fibroids of low signal intensity (*white circles*). The tumor extends into the upper vagina. (*B*) Sagittal T1-weighted fat-saturation post-gadolinium image shows enhancement of the cervical mass. (*C*) On the axial T2-weighted image the normal T2 low signal intensity fibrous stroma is absent (*arrows*) and there is contour irregularity suspicious for parametrial invasion.

and CT had a low sensitivity (42% for CT, 53% for MR imaging) but high specificity (82% for CT, 74% for MR imaging) and NPV (84% for CT, 85% for MR imaging).[45]

Areas where imaging can potentially impact on patient management are the evaluation of young patients for possible trachelectomy, assessment of tumor volume, and tumor response to therapy.

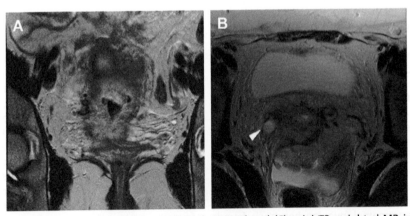

Fig. 6. Cervical carcinoma in a 45-year-old woman. (*A*) Coronal and (*B*) axial T2-weighted MR imaging shows a bulky heterogeneous cervical mass with invasion of the cervical stroma. There is dilatation of the adjacent distal right ureter (*arrowhead*) secondary to parametrial invasion.

Trachelectomy involves resection of the cervix and upper 1- to 2-cm of vagina and parametrium, with preservation of the uterine corpus for future fertility in patients of reproductive age with stage I cervical cancer.[49] The uterine corpus is incised from the cervix approximately 5 mm below the internal os, the resected cervix is assessed for a tumor-free margin, and the uterine body is sutured to the upper vagina. Location of the cervical tumor margin relative to the internal os and lower uterine segment myometrium is helpful in determining if the patient is a candidate for this procedure (**Fig. 7**). A waist in the uterine contour, differences in the signal intensity of the cervical stroma relative to the myometrium, and location of the uterine vessels have been used to define the location of the internal os on imaging.[50] A study by 2 experienced readers found that the internal os was visible on MR imaging in most patients, with good interobserver variability for estimating the distance of the tumor from the internal os.[51] High sensitivity and specificity of MR imaging for tumor involvement of the internal os as compared with surgery has also been reported.[44] Retrospective analysis of MR imaging in 150 patients found a sensitivity of 90%, specificity of 98%, PPV of 86%, and NPV of 98% for tumor extension to internal os.[43]

In addition to staging, the appearance of the cervical tumor on imaging may be helpful in predicting patient response to nonsurgical therapy and outcome. Tumor volume before and after treatment can be calculated from the largest-diameter measurements on multiplanar images and may help as a prognostic indicator in these patients.[52]

Dynamic contrast-enhanced MR imaging is also an exciting new method to assess tumor angiogenesis and perfusion of cervical cancer before and after therapy. The contrast agent diffuses into the extravascular space, with no linear relationship between the concentration of gadolinium and the resultant tissue signal. The degree of enhancement is related to a combination of blood flow, vascular permeability, and volume of extracellular space. Semiquantitative parameters obtained by plotting tissue signal intensity over time depend on machine and imaging parameters. Quantitative analysis using pharmacokinetic modeling provides parameters such as the transfer constant between blood plasma and the extravascular extracellular space, and the volume of the extravascular extracellular space.[53] Increased tumor enhancement suggests increased vascularity and oxygenation, which may indicate increased radiosensitivity and delivery of therapeutic drugs. Dynamic contrast-enhanced MR imaging has been performed in patients with cervical cancer before and during radiation and has been shown to predict response to therapy and disease-free survival.[54–58]

DWI also has the potential to demonstrate the primary tumor in cervical cancer and response to treatment.[59,60] Cervical cancer has a lower ADC value than that of the normal epithelium. ADC values have been noted to increase with treatment.[59–61]

Role of Imaging for Assessment of Nodal and Distant Metastases, and Recurrence

Nodal disease is not assessed in the clinical FIGO staging system but does influence patient prognosis. Tumor can initially spread to the external iliac, internal iliac, and presacral nodes, followed

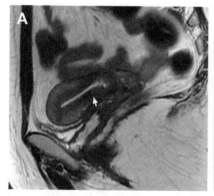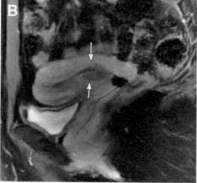

Fig. 7. Cervical carcinoma in a 35-year-old woman who was initially considered for trachelectomy. (*A*) Sagittal T2-weighted and (*B*) sagittal T1-weighted fat-saturation post-gadolinium MR imaging shows endocervical tumor up to the internal os. There is abnormal signal intensity (*arrows*) in the anterior cervical stroma with extension to the junctional zone of the anterior lower uterine segment. Trachelectomy was attempted but the cervical margin was positive for tumor, and the patient underwent hysterectomy.

by the common iliac and para-aortic nodes.[62] The extent of lymphadenectomy and radiation field may need to be increased if para-aortic nodes are suspicious for metastatic involvement. As for other tumors, findings suggestive of nodal tumor include a short-axis diameter greater than 1 cm and the presence of necrosis. Size criteria are, however, not reliable.[63] In the ACRIN/GOG trial, sensitivity was low for both MR imaging and CT (37% and 31%) but specificity was high (94% and 86%).[45] The prediction of nodal involvement on MR imaging was higher than for CT when combined with results for tumor size.[47] A 10-year review of 150 patients with early-stage cervical cancer at a single institution also found similar sensitivity and specificity for nodal metastases with MR imaging.[43] Sensitivity slightly improves but specificity decreases when the short-axis diameter cutoff for distinguishing normal from abnormal nodes is decreased from 1 cm to 0.5 cm.[44] A meta-analysis of 57 MR imaging and/or CT articles reported a sensitivity of 60% for MR imaging and 43% for CT with equivalent specificity.[38] Another meta-analysis that included PET found that on a per-patient basis, PET or PET/CT had higher sensitivity (82%) compared with CT (50%) or MR imaging (56%), with all 3 having specificities of greater than 90%. On a region or node based basis, sensitivity was in a similar range with 54% for PET, 52% for CT, and 38% for MR imaging.[64] The addition of DWI or lymph node contrast agents to MR imaging has been suggested.[65] Ultrasmall superparamagnetic iron oxide (USPIO) particles are taken up by macrophages in nodes resulting in a loss of signal on gradient echo sequences. However, in metastatic nodes there is replacement of the normal nodal architecture by tumor, resulting in diminished macrophages and lack of significant signal loss. This method can increase the sensitivity of MR imaging for identifying nodal metastases.[66]

Recurrent cervical cancer occurs mainly in the pelvis in the vaginal vault, parametrium, and pelvic side wall. Distant metastases occur in the peritoneum, liver, adrenal glands, lungs, and bones.[66] Local recurrence is better evaluated with MR imaging, whereas CT is used in search of distant sites. Posttreatment changes can be difficult to distinguish from residual or recurrent tumor, as inflammation can show increased signal on T2-weighted images and enhancement similar to tumor.

OVARIAN CARCINOMA

Ovarian carcinoma is the second most frequent gynecologic malignancy in the United States with approximately 20,000 new cases annually. About two-thirds of patients present with advanced FIGO Stage III or IV disease. Ovarian cancer accounts for a greater number of deaths than all other gynecologic malignancies.[1,67] The World Health Organization subdivides ovarian tumors into 3 main types based on the cell of origin: epithelial, sex-cord stromal, and germ cell tumors.[68] Epithelial tumors account for approximately 90% of ovarian cancers and can have serous, mucinous, endometrioid, clear cell, and undifferentiated histologies.[69,70] Serous carcinoma represents approximately 80% of all ovarian cancers and is histologically graded as low or high grade. Low-grade serous carcinomas arise from borderline tumors whereas high-grade tumors do not have a definite precursor lesion, are more frequent, and have a poorer prognosis. Borderline tumors lack stromal invasion and occur at a younger age group than invasive cancer. Primary ovarian mucinous carcinoma is uncommon and is diagnosed after excluding metastatic disease to the ovary.

Role of Imaging in Primary Tumor Assessment

Imaging is used to characterize an adnexal mass and assess for metastatic disease following the diagnosis of malignancy. US is the first-line approach for lesion characterization, with MR imaging a problem-solving tool. CT or MR imaging can be used to stage patients for metastatic disease. Adnexal lesions are common findings on imaging procedures, and the key is to distinguish benign from potentially malignant lesions.

Functional cysts occur in premenopausal women, and cysts are also seen in approximately 20% of postmenopausal women. Short-term follow-up imaging is helpful to distinguish functional from pathologic cystic lesions. Benign lesions include corpus luteum cysts, endometriomas, dermoids, and hydrosalpinx. Feature analysis is used to determine the likelihood of a benign lesion that need only be followed, or of indeterminate or malignant lesions that require resection.[67,71] Simple cysts are anechoic on US with increased through transmission and no internal soft tissue. Sonographic, CT, and MR imaging criteria suspicious for malignancy include the presence of a vascular soft tissue component. This component can further consist of septations greater than 3 mm in thickness, papillary projections, or nodules (**Figs. 8–10**).[72] A retracted blood clot, fibrin strands, and dermoid plug are benign causes of soft tissue nodularity. Assessment of nodule echogenicity and color Doppler imaging for internal vascularity are helpful.[72,73] Combining

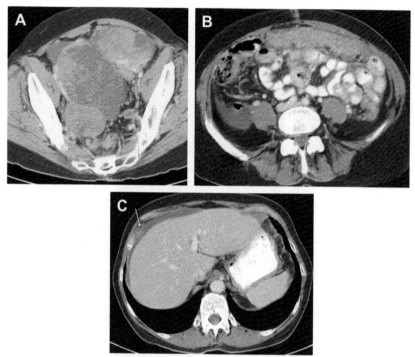

Fig. 8. High-grade serous ovarian carcinoma in a 70-year-old woman with a pelvic mass and elevated serum CA125 level. Intravenous and oral contrast-enhanced axial CT images demonstrate (*A*) bilateral heterogeneous enhancing adnexal masses in the pelvis, (*B*) anterior omental cake and small amount of ascites in the mid-abdomen, and (*C*) a peritoneal deposit (*arrow*) adjacent to the liver.

Doppler with gray-scale imaging improves the diagnostic assessment of ovarian lesions. A meta-analysis of 46 studies compared the relative utility of gray-scale imaging, color Doppler, and Doppler flow analysis for interrogating adnexal masses, and found that the combination of these methods was more powerful than their individual use.[74] Although US and MR imaging are both highly sensitive for adnexal lesions, MR imaging is more specific for characterization of fat and blood products. MR imaging can also evaluate solid components in large lesions that may be difficult to entirely visualize on US. In a study of 103 women with sonographic features worrisome for adnexal malignancy, MR imaging and US both had a sensitivity of greater than 80% for malignancy but the specificity for MR imaging, 84%, was much higher than for US, 59%, due to the ability of MR imaging to accurately define benign lesions such as dermoid, endometrioma, and fibroid.[67,75] Increased specificity can affect patient management and may obviate the need for surgery.[76] A meta-analysis showed that in a patient with a sonographically indeterminate adnexal lesion, the posttest probability of malignancy increased with the addition of MR imaging and, to a lesser extent, CT.[77] In a review of 143 patients

with CT and histopathology, features suspicious for malignancy in cystic lesions included multilocularity, irregular wall thickening, and soft tissue nodules, while unilocular homogeneous lesions with thin walls and smooth contour tended to be benign.[71] Secondary findings of implants, ascites, and other metastases also aid in distinguishing malignant from benign lesions.

In addition to the traditional feature analysis method of evaluating adnexal lesions, there have been reports on applying contrast-enhanced US and dynamic contrast-enhanced MR imaging for these masses. In sonographic studies of patients who were imaged for 3 to 5 minutes after contrast injection, malignancies have had a slower washout of contrast than benign lesions.[78–80] The development of diagnostic criteria for the kinetics of contrast enhancement may increase the specificity of US for adnexal malignancies.[80] Malignancies have a faster time to peak and greater enhancement on dynamic contrast-enhanced MR imaging than benign lesions.[81] A report correlating dynamic MR imaging with histology found a positive correlation between the slope of the enhancement curve and tumor expression of vascular endothelial growth factor receptor, which plays a role in angiogenesis.[81] DWI also provides tissue perfusion

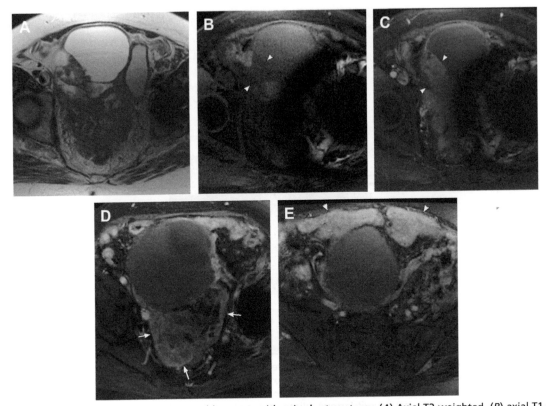

Fig. 9. Ovarian carcinoma in an 80-year-old woman with prior hysterectomy. (A) Axial T2-weighted, (B) axial T1-weighted fat-saturation precontrast, and (C) axial T1-weighted fat-saturation post-gadolinium MR imaging show a complex cystic ovarian mass with an enhancing solid component (*arrowheads*). (D and E) Axial T1-weighted fat-saturation post-gadolinium images at more superior levels demonstrate enhancing serosal disease involving the bowel (*arrows* in D) and omental tissue (*arrowheads* in E). Susceptibility artifact from left hip replacement is noted in the left pelvis.

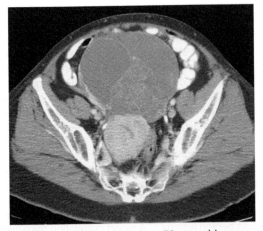

Fig. 10. Ovarian metastasis in a 50-year-old woman. Intravenous and oral contrast-enhanced axial CT through the pelvis shows a multiseptate midline cystic mass, histologically proven as metastasis from a mucinous adenocarcinoma of the pancreatic tail (not shown).

information at low b values, and the vascular signal intensity has been preliminarily investigated in the primary tumor and abdominal metastases of advanced epithelial ovarian cancer.[82]

Ovarian carcinoma is staged surgically with exploratory laparotomy, oophorectomy, hysterectomy, omentectomy, and peritoneal washings, as well as inspection and resection of abdominal and pelvic implants (**Table 3**). The goal of surgery is to optimally debulk patients to deposits of residual disease less than 1 cm in size. Tumor spreads to the contralateral ovary, uterus, and peritoneum. Cells are carried up into the abdomen by the peritoneal fluid that normally circulates from the pelvis to the abdomen along a clockwise pathway—initially to the right paracolic gutter, the right upper quadrant around the liver and diaphragm, and thence to the greater omentum and left paracolic gutter. Implants are therefore usually found in the cul-de-sac, paracolic and subphrenic spaces, greater omentum, and on the surfaces of the liver, bowel, and spleen.[68,70,73,83,84] Preoperative CT or MR

Table 3 FIGO staging of ovarian carcinoma	
I	Tumor limited to ovary
IA	Tumor limited to one ovary with intact capsule and no tumor on ovarian surface. No tumor cells in ascites or peritoneal washings
IB	Tumor limited to both ovaries with intact capsule and no tumor on ovarian surface. No tumor cells in ascites or peritoneal washings
IC	Tumor limited to one or both ovaries with: ruptured capsule or tumor on ovarian surface or tumor cells in ascites or peritoneal washings
II	Ovarian tumor with pelvic extension and/or implants
IIA	Extension and/or implants on fallopian tube(s) and/or uterus No tumor cells in ascites or peritoneal washings
IIB	Extension to and/or implants on other pelvic soft tissues No tumor cells in ascites or peritoneal washings
IIC	Extension to and/or implants on pelvic soft tissues with tumor cells in ascites or peritoneal washings
III	Peritoneal metastases outside the pelvis
IIIA	Microscopic peritoneal metastasis beyond pelvis
IIIB	Macroscopic ($\leq$2 cm) peritoneal metastasis beyond pelvis
IIIC	Macroscopic (>2 cm) peritoneal metastasis beyond pelvis and/or metastasis to regional nodes
IV	Distant metastasis

Note: Liver capsule metastases are Stage III and liver parenchymal metastases are Stage IV.

From Mironov S, Akin O, Pandit-Taskar N, et al. Ovarian cancer. Radiol Clin North Am 2007;45:56.

imaging can be used to determine the extent of disease.[68] Metastatic implants appear as discrete nodules, masses, nodularity, or plaque-like thickening on the surface of viscera, and can enhance.[85,86] Implants on the liver and spleen can cause scalloping of the surface. Protrusion of the implant into the liver with irregularity of the interface suggests invasion of the parenchyma by tumor, which may require more extensive resection.[87]

MR imaging and CT perform similarly in the preoperative staging of ovarian carcinoma.[75,84,88,89] Staging is primarily done with CT

because of its shorter imaging time and ready availability. Sensitivity is higher for lesions larger than 1 to 2 cm as well as for those surrounded by ascitic fluid. CT is more sensitive than MR imaging for calcified implants. In a study on 64 patients scanned with CT slice thickness of 5 to 10 mm, sensitivity was lower for subcentimeter implants, 25% to 50%, as compared with overall sensitivity of 85% to 93% for peritoneal disease.[90] Thinner slices are possible with current MDCT scanners, and multiplanar images have an incremental value over axial images for detecting metastases.[91] Sensitivity and specificity on CT and MR imaging can also depend on the lesion location, paracolic gutters versus diaphragm.[86,91] Small implants on the bowel are particularly difficult to detect with CT and MR imaging but can have greater conspicuity on PET/CT. A recent study on 133 patients with ovarian masses found a sensitivity of 94% and specificity of 71% for CT or MR imaging for diagnosis of extraovarian abdominopelvic metastases, whereas PET/CT had a higher specificity of 83% for a similar sensitivity.[92] The addition of the DWI sequence to MR imaging improved the sensitivity for peritoneal metastases in 34 patients with ovarian and non-ovarian cancers from 73% to 90% while specificity remained similar, at 90%.[93]

Pelvic sites of disease are easily assessed and debulked at surgery. However, resection of tumors in the upper abdomen can be more difficult, and preoperative imaging can help in the surgical planning for locations such as the lesser sac, porta hepatis, diaphragm, and mesentery. Parenchymal liver metastases also need to be distinguished from surface implants (**Figs. 11** and **12**). In a study of 137 women with a new diagnosis of ovarian carcinoma, CT and MR imaging were equally

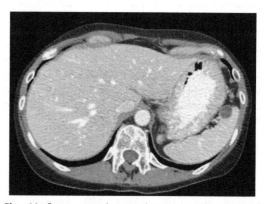

Fig. 11. Serous ovarian carcinoma in a 60-year-old woman. Intravenous and oral contrast-enhanced axial CT through the upper abdomen shows a cystic splenic surface metastatic implant.

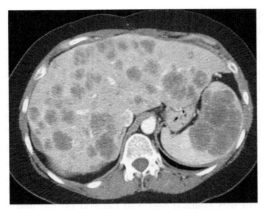

Fig. 12. Ovarian carcinoma in a 50-year-old woman. Intravenous and oral contrast-enhanced axial CT through the upper abdomen demonstrates multiple parenchymal liver and splenic metastases.

able to predict which patients were less likely to have effective cytoreduction, with sensitivity, specificity, PPV, and NPV of 76%, 99%, 94%, and 96%, respectively.[94]

Role of Imaging for Assessment of Nodal and Distant Metastases and Recurrence

The peritoneal route of dissemination is the most common for ovarian cancer, with lymphatic and hematogenous metastases being less common. Pelvic nodal metastases occur following tumor spread via the broad ligament. Para-aortic nodes can be involved by tumor spread along the gonadal vessels.[70] Supradiaphragmatic lymph node metastases can be also found.[68] Size criteria are used to assess nodes similar to other malignancies. Hematogenous metastases are least common and as a rule involve the liver, lung, and pleura.[70,73] Treated patients are followed by serial CA125 assays and CT or MR imaging of the abdomen and pelvis. PET/CT can be helpful in the presence of rising tumor markers with no obvious disease on CT. Recurrence occurs typically in the peritoneal cavity, lymph nodes, abdominal viscera, and thorax,[95,96] and can be identified for preoperative planning. In a series of 36 patients with recurrent ovarian cancer, the presence of pelvic side-wall invasion at CT was predictive of suboptimal secondary cytoreduction.[88]

SUMMARY

Initial assessment of patients with symptoms suspicious for gynecologic malignancy is performed with US, using MR imaging as a problem-solving tool for indeterminate lesions. Local staging of uterine malignancies is primarily done with MR imaging whereas ovarian malignancies are typically staged by CT. Morphologic imaging features are used primarily for distinguishing benign from malignant gynecologic masses and for evaluating potential metastatic disease. Newer tools such as DWI and dynamic contrast-enhanced imaging may result in improved lesion characterization and staging.

REFERENCES

1. American Cancer Society. Cancer facts and figures. Atlanta (GA): American Cancer Society; 2009.
2. Mendivil A, Schuler KM, Gehrig PA. Non-endometrioid adenocarcinoma of the uterine corpus: a review of selected histological subtypes. Cancer Control 2009;16:46–52.
3. Prat J, Gallardo A, Cuatrecasas M, et al. Endometrial carcinoma: pathology and genetics. Pathology 2007;39:72–87.
4. Peungjesada S, Bhosale PR, Balachandran A, et al. Magnetic resonance imaging of endometrial carcinoma. J Comput Assist Tomogr 2009;33:601–8.
5. Goldstein RB, Bree RL, Benson CB, et al. Evaluation of the woman with postmenopausal bleeding: Society of Radiologists in Ultrasound-Sponsored Consensus Conference statement. J Ultrasound Med 2001;20:1025–36.
6. Smith-Bindman R, Kerlikowske K, Feldstein VA, et al. Endovaginal ultrasound to exclude endometrial cancer and other endometrial abnormalities. JAMA 1998;280:1510–7.
7. Laifer-Narin S, Ragavendra N, Parmenter EK, et al. False-normal appearance of the endometrium on conventional transvaginal sonography: comparison with saline hysterosonography. AJR Am J Roentgenol 2002;178:129–33.
8. Bree RL, Bowerman RA, Bohm-Velez M, et al. US evaluation of the uterus in patients with postmenopausal bleeding: a positive effect on diagnostic decision making. Radiology 2000;216:260–4.
9. Davidson KG, Dubinsky TJ. Ultrasonographic evaluation of the endometrium in postmenopausal vaginal bleeding. Radiol Clin North Am 2003;41:769–80.
10. Dubinsky TJ, Stroehlein K, Abu-Ghazzeh Y, et al. Prediction of benign and malignant endometrial disease: hysterosonographic-pathologic correlation. Radiology 1999;210:393–7.
11. Frei KA, Kinkel K. Staging endometrial cancer: role of magnetic resonance imaging. J Magn Reson Imaging 2001;13:850–5.
12. Manfredi R, Gui B, Maresca G, et al. Endometrial cancer: magnetic resonance imaging. Abdom Imaging 2005;30:626–36.
13. Saez F, Urresola A, Larena JA, et al. Endometrial carcinoma: assessment of myometrial invasion with plain and gadolinium-enhanced MR imaging. J Magn Reson Imaging 2000;12:460–6.

14. Creasman W. Revised FIGO staging for carcinoma of the endometrium. Int J Gynaecol Obstet 2009; 105:109.

15. Manfredi R, Mirk P, Maresca G, et al. Local-regional staging of endometrial carcinoma: role of MR imaging in surgical planning. Radiology 2004;231:372–8.

16. Chung HH, Kang SB, Cho JY, et al. Accuracy of MR imaging for the prediction of myometrial invasion of endometrial carcinoma. Gynecol Oncol 2007;104: 654–9.

17. Nakao Y, Yokoyama M, Hara K, et al. MR imaging in endometrial carcinoma as a diagnostic tool for the absence of myometrial invasion. Gynecol Oncol 2006;102:343–7.

18. Félix A, Cunha TM. Preoperative assessment of deep myometrial and cervical invasion in endometrial carcinoma: comparison of magnetic resonance imaging and histopathologic evaluation. J Obstet Gynaecol 2007;27:65–70.

19. Sala E, Crawford R, Senior E, et al. Added value of dynamic contrast-enhanced magnetic resonance imaging in predicting advanced stage disease in patients with endometrial carcinoma. Int J Gynecol Cancer 2009;19:141–6.

20. Utsunomiya D, Notsute S, Hayashida Y, et al. Endometrial carcinoma in adenomyosis: assessment of myometrial invasion on T2-weighted spin-echo and gadolinium-enhanced T1-weighted images. AJR Am J Roentgenol 2004;182:399–404.

21. Frei KA, Kinkel K, Bonᵗl HM, et al. Prediction of deep myometrial invasion in patients with endometrial cancer: clinical utility of contrast-enhanced MR imaging-a meta-analysis and Bayesian analysis. Radiology 2000;216:444–9.

22. Shen SH, Chiou YY, Wang JH, et al. Diffusion-weighted single-shot echo-planar imaging with parallel technique in assessment of endometrial cancer. AJR Am J Roentgenol 2008;190:481–8.

23. Tamai K, Koyama T, Saga T, et al. Diffusion-weighted MR imaging of uterine endometrial cancer. J Magn Reson Imaging 2007;26:682–7.

24. Inada Y, Matsuki M, Nakai G, et al. Body diffusion-weighted MR imaging of uterine endometrial cancer: is it helpful in the detection of cancer in nonenhanced MR imaging? Eur J Radiol 2009;70:122–7.

25. Takeuchi M, Matsuzaki K, Nishitani H. Diffusion-weighted magnetic resonance imaging of endometrial cancer: differentiation from benign endometrial lesions and preoperative assessment of myometrial invasion. Acta Radiol 2009;50:947–53.

26. Rechichi G, Galimberti S, Signorelli M, et al. Myometrial invasion in endometrial cancer: diagnostic performance of diffusion-weighted MR imaging at 1.5-T. Eur Radiol 2010;20:754–62.

27. Kinkel K, Kaji Y, Yu KK, et al. Radiologic staging in patients with endometrial cancer: a meta-analysis. Radiology 1999;212:711–8.

28. Ozdemir S, Celik C, Emlik D, et al. Assessment of myometrial invasion in endometrial cancer by transvaginal sonography, Doppler ultrasonography, magnetic resonance imaging and frozen section. Int J Gynecol Cancer 2009;19:1085–90.

29. Alcázar JL, Galván R, Albela S, et al. Assessing myometrial infiltration by endometrial cancer: uterine virtual navigation with three-dimensional US. Radiology 2009;250:776–83.

30. Song Y, Yang J, Liu Z, et al. Preoperative evaluation of endometrial carcinoma by contrast-enhanced ultrasonography. BJOG 2009;116:294–8 [discussion: 298–9].

31. Hardesty LA, Sumkin JH, Hakim C, et al. The ability of helical CT to preoperatively stage endometrial carcinoma. AJR Am J Roentgenol 2001;176:603–6.

32. Tsili AC, Tsampoulas C, Dalkalitsis N, et al. Local staging of endometrial carcinoma: role of multidetector CT. Eur Radiol 2008;18:1043–8.

33. Chi DS, Barakat RR, Palayekar MJ, et al. The incidence of pelvic lymph node metastasis by FIGO staging for patients with adequately surgically staged endometrial adenocarcinoma of endometrioid histology. Int J Gynecol Cancer 2008;18:269–73.

34. Celik C, Ozdemir S, Esen H, et al. The clinical value of preoperative and intraoperative assessments in the management of endometrial cancer. Int J Gynecol Cancer 2010;20:358–62.

35. Namimoto T, Awai K, Nakaura T, et al. Role of diffusion-weighted imaging in the diagnosis of gynecological diseases. Eur Radiol 2009;19:745–60.

36. Lin G, Ng KK, Chang CJ, et al. Myometrial invasion in endometrial cancer: diagnostic accuracy of diffusion-weighted 3.0-T MR imaging—initial experience. Radiology 2009;250:784–92.

37. Ozsarlak O, Tjalma W, Schepens E, et al. The correlation of preoperative CT, MR imaging, and clinical staging (FIGO) with histopathology findings in primary cervical carcinoma. Eur Radiol 2003;13: 2338–45.

38. Bipat S, Glas AS, van der Velden J, et al. Computed tomography and magnetic resonance imaging in staging of uterine cervical carcinoma: a systematic review. Gynecol Oncol 2003;91:59–66.

39. Seki H, Azumi R, Kimura M, et al. Stromal invasion by carcinoma of the cervix: assessment by dynamic MR imaging. AJR Am J Roentgenol 1997;168:1579–85.

40. deSouza NM, Dina R, McIndoe GA, et al. Cervical cancer: value of an endovaginal coil magnetic resonance imaging technique in detecting small volume disease and assessing parametrial extension. Gynecol Oncol 2006;102:80–5.

41. Hancke K, Heilmann V, Straka P, et al. Pretreatment staging of cervical cancer: is imaging better than palpation?: role of CT and MRI in preoperative staging of cervical cancer: single institution results for 255 patients. Ann Surg Oncol 2008;15:2856–61.

42. Choi SH, Kim SH, Choi HJ, et al. Preoperative magnetic resonance imaging staging of uterine cervical carcinoma: results of prospective study. J Comput Assist Tomogr 2004;28:620–7.

43. Sahdev A, Sohaib SA, Wenaden AE, et al. The performance of magnetic resonance imaging in early cervical carcinoma: a long-term experience. Int J Gynecol Cancer 2007;17:629–36.

44. Manfredi R, Gui B, Giovanzana A, et al. Localized cervical cancer (stage <IIB): accuracy of MR imaging in planning less extensive surgery. Radiol Med 2009;114:960–75.

45. Hricak H, Gatsonis C, Chi DS, et al. Role of imaging in pretreatment evaluation of early invasive cervical cancer: results of the intergroup study American College of Radiology Imaging Network 6651-Gynecologic Oncology Group 183. J Clin Oncol 2005; 23:9329–37.

46. Mitchell DG, Snyder B, Coakley F, et al. Early invasive cervical cancer: tumor delineation by magnetic resonance imaging, computed tomography, and clinical examination, verified by pathologic results, in the ACRIN 6651/GOG 183 Intergroup Study. J Clin Oncol 2006;24:5687–94.

47. Mitchell DG, Snyder B, Coakley F, et al. Early invasive cervical cancer: MRI and CT predictors of lymphatic metastases in the ACRIN 6651/GOG 183 intergroup study. Gynecol Oncol 2009;112: 95–103.

48. Hricak H, Gatsonis C, Coakley FV, et al. Early invasive cervical cancer: CT and MR imaging in preoperative evaluation—ACRIN/GOG comparative study of diagnostic performance and interobserver variability. Radiology 2007;245:491–8.

49. Abu-Rustum NR, Sonoda Y, Black D, et al. Fertility-sparing radical abdominal trachelectomy for cervical carcinoma: technique and review of the literature. Gynecol Oncol 2006;103:807–13.

50. Peppercorn PD, Jeyarajah AR, Woolas R, et al. Role of MR imaging in the selection of patients with early cervical carcinoma for fertility-preserving surgery: initial experience. Radiology 1999;212:395–9.

51. Bipat S, van den Berg RA, van der Velden J, et al. The role of magnetic resonance imaging in determining the proximal extension of early stage cervical cancer to the internal os. Eur J Radiol 2009. [Epub ahead of print].

52. Lee DW, Kim YT, Kim JH, et al. Clinical significance of tumor volume and lymph node involvement assessed by MRI in stage IIB cervical cancer patients treated with concurrent chemoradiation therapy. J Gynecol Oncol 2010;21:18–23.

53. Tofts PS, Brix G, Buckley DL, et al. Estimating kinetic parameters from dynamic contrast-enhanced T(1)-weighted MRI of a diffusible tracer: standardized quantities and symbols. J Magn Reson Imaging 1999;10:223–32.

54. Yuh WT, Mayr NA, Jarjoura D, et al. Predicting control of primary tumor and survival by DCE MRI during early therapy in cervical cancer. Invest Radiol 2009;44:343–50.

55. Mayr NA, Wang JZ, Zhang D, et al. Longitudinal changes in tumor perfusion pattern during the radiation therapy course and its clinical impact in cervical cancer. Int J Radiat Oncol Biol Phys 2010; 77:502–8.

56. Zahra MA, Tan LT, Priest AN, et al. Semiquantitative and quantitative dynamic contrast-enhanced magnetic resonance imaging measurements predict radiation response in cervix cancer. Int J Radiat Oncol Biol Phys 2009;74:766–73.

57. Semple SI, Harry VN, Parkin DE, et al. A combined pharmacokinetic and radiologic assessment of dynamic contrast-enhanced magnetic resonance imaging predicts response to chemoradiation in locally advanced cervical cancer. Int J Radiat Oncol Biol Phys 2009;75:611–7.

58. Donaldson SB, Buckley DL, O'Connor JP. Enhancing fraction measured using dynamic contrast-enhanced MRI predicts disease-free survival in patients with carcinoma of the cervix. Br J Cancer 2010;102:23–6.

59. Messiou C, Morgan VA, De Silva SS, et al. Diffusion weighted imaging of the uterus: regional ADC variation with oral contraceptive usage and comparison with cervical cancer. Acta Radiol 2009;50:696–701.

60. Liu Y, Bai R, Sun H, et al. Diffusion-weighted imaging in predicting and monitoring the response of uterine cervical cancer to combined chemoradiation. Clin Radiol 2009;64:1067–74.

61. Payne GS, Schmidt M, Morgan VA, et al. Evaluation of magnetic resonance diffusion and spectroscopy measurements as predictive biomarkers in stage 1 cervical cancer. Gynecol Oncol 2010;116(2):246–52.

62. Park JM, Charnsangavej C, Yoshimitsu K, et al. Pathways of nodal metastasis from pelvic tumors: CT demonstration. Radiographics 1994;14(6):1309–21.

63. Yang WT, Man Lam WW, Yu MY, et al. Comparison of dynamic helical CT and dynamic MR imaging in the evaluation of pelvic lymph nodes in cervical carcinoma. AJR Am J Roentgenol 2000;175:759–66.

64. Choi HJ, Ju W, Myung SK, et al. Diagnostic performance of computer tomography, magnetic resonance imaging, and positron emission tomography or positron emission tomography/computer tomography for detection of metastatic lymph nodes in patients with cervical cancer: meta-analysis. Cancer Sci 2010;101:1471–9.

65. Lin G, Ho KC, Wang JJ, et al. Detection of lymph node metastasis in cervical and uterine cancers by diffusion-weighted magnetic resonance imaging at 3T. J Magn Reson Imaging 2008;28:128–35.

66. Sala E, Wakely S, Senior E, et al. MRI of malignant neoplasms of the uterine corpus and cervix. AJR Am J Roentgenol 2007;188:1577–87.

67. Rieber A, Nussle K, Stohr I, et al. Preoperative diagnosis of ovarian tumors with MR imaging: comparison with transvaginal sonography, positron emission tomography, and histologic findings AJR. Am J Roentgenol 2001;177:123–9.

68. Edge SB, Byrd DR, Compton CC, et al, editors. AJCC cancer staging handbook. 7th edition. New York: Springer; 2010.

69. Iyer VR, Lee SI. MRI, CT and PET/CT for ovarian cancer detection and adnexal lesion characterization. AJR Am J Roentgenol 2010;194:311–21.

70. Mironov S, Akin O, Pandit-Taskar N, et al. Ovarian cancer. Radiol Clin North Am 2007;45:149–66.

71. Zhang J, Mironov S, Hricak H, et al. Characterization of adnexal masses using feature analysis at contrast-enhanced helical computed tomography. J Comput Assist Tomogr 2008;32:533–40.

72. Brown DL, Dudiak KM, Laing FC. Adnexal masses: US characterization and reporting. Radiology 2010; 254:342–54.

73. Shaaban A, Rezvani M. Ovarian cancer: detection and radiologic staging. Clin Obstet Gynecol 2009; 52:73–93.

74. Kinkel K, Hricak H, Lu Ying, et al. US characterization of ovarian masses: a meta-analysis. Radiology 2000;217:803–11.

75. Kurtz AB, Tsimikas JV, Tempany CM, et al. Diagnosis and staging of ovarian cancer: comparative values of Doppler and conventional US, CT, and MR imaging correlated with surgery and histopathologic analysis—report of the Radiology Diagnostic Oncology Group. Radiology 1999;212:19–27.

76. Spencer JA, Forstner R, Cunha TM, et al. ESUR Female Imaging Sub-Committee. ESUR guidelines for MR imaging of the sonographically indeterminate adnexal mass: an algorithmic approach. Eur Radiol 2010;20:25–35.

77. Kinkel K, Lu Y, Mehdizade A, et al. Indeterminate ovarian mass at US: incremental value of second imaging test for characterization—meta-analysis and Bayesian analysis. Radiology 2005;236:85–94.

78. Ordén MR, Jurvelin JS, Kirkinen PP. Kinetics of a US contrast agent in benign and malignant adnexal tumors. Radiology 2003;226:405–10.

79. Marret H, Sauget S, Giraudeau B, et al. Contrast-enhanced sonography helps in discrimination of benign from malignant adnexal masses. J Ultrasound Med 2004;23:1629–39.

80. Fleischer AC, Lyshchik A, Jones HW 3rd, et al. Diagnostic parameters to differentiate benign from malignant ovarian masses with contrast-enhanced transvaginal sonography. J Ultrasound Med 2009; 28:1273–780.

81. Thomassin-Naggara I, Bazot M, Daraï E, et al. Epithelial ovarian tumors: value of dynamic contrast-enhanced MR imaging and correlation with tumor angiogenesis. Radiology 2008;248:148–59.

82. Sala E, Priest AN, Kataoka M, et al. Apparent diffusion coefficient and vascular signal fraction measurements with magnetic resonance imaging: feasibility in metastatic ovarian cancer at 3 Tesla: technical development. Eur Radiol 2010;20:491–6.

83. Coakley FV, Hricak H. Imaging of peritoneal and mesenteric disease: key concepts for the clinical radiologist. Clin Radiol 1999;54:563–74.

84. Tempany CMC, Zou KH, Silverman SG, et al. Staging of advanced ovarian cancer: comparison of imaging modalities—report from the Radiological Diagnostic Oncology Group. Radiology 2000;215:761–7.

85. Forstner R, Hricak H, Occhipinti KA, et al. Ovarian cancer: staging with CT and MR imaging. Radiology 1995;197:619–26.

86. Ricke J, Sehouli J, Hach C, et al. Prospective evaluation of contrast-enhanced MRI in the depiction of peritoneal spread in primary or recurrent ovarian cancer. Eur Radiol 2003;13:943–9.

87. Akin O, Sala E, Moskowitz CS, et al. Perihepatic metastases from ovarian cancer: sensitivity and specificity of CT for the detection of metastases with and those without liver parenchymal invasion. Radiology 2008;248:511–7.

88. Funt SA, Hricak H, Abu-Rustum N, et al. Role of CT in the management of recurrent ovarian cancer. AJR Am J Roentgenol 2004;182:393–8.

89. Pecorelli S. Revised FIGO staging for carcinoma of the vulva, cervix, and endometrium. Int J Gynaecol Obstet 2009;105:103–4.

90. Coakley FV, Choi PH, Gougoutas CA, et al. Peritoneal metastases: detection with spiral CT in patients with ovarian cancer. Radiology 2002;223:495–9.

91. Pannu HK, Horton KM, Fishman EK. Thin section dual-phase multidetector-row computed tomography detection of peritoneal metastases in gynecologic cancers. J Comput Assist Tomogr 2003;27:333–40.

92. Nam EJ, Yun MJ, Oh YT, et al. Diagnosis and staging of primary ovarian cancer: correlation between PET/CT, Doppler US, and CT or MRI. Gynecol Oncol 2010;116:389–94.

93. Low RN, Sebrechts CP, Barone RM, et al. Diffusion-weighted MRI of peritoneal tumors: comparison with conventional MRI and surgical and histopathologic findings—a feasibility study. AJR Am J Roentgenol 2009;193:461–70.

94. Qayyum A, Coakley FV, Westphalen AC, et al. Role of CT and MR imaging in predicting optimal cytoreduction of newly diagnosed primary epithelial ovarian cancer. Gynecol Oncol 2005;96:301–6.

95. Park CM, Kim SH, Kim SH, et al. Recurrent ovarian malignancy: patterns and spectrum of imaging findings. Abdom Imaging 2003;28:404–15.

96. Sahdev A, Hughes JH, Barwick T, et al. Computed tomography features of recurrent ovarian carcinoma according to time to relapse. Acta Radiol 2007;48:1038–44.

Imaging the Normal and Abnormal Anatomy of the Female Pelvis Using ^{18}F FDG-PET/CT, Including Pitfalls and Artifacts

Einat Even-Sapir, MD, PhD

KEYWORDS

- ^{18}F FDG uptake • Female reproductive system
- Cancer • PET/CT

Imaging by ^{18}F fluorodeoxyglucose (FDG)-PET has been introduced in the imaging algorithm of various oncologic diseases. Accurate interpretation of PET images often requires separation between abnormal ^{18}F FDG activity in malignant lesions and physiologic uptake. In the pelvis, the latter can be detected in the gastrointestinal and urinary tracts. In the reproductive age, the endometrium and ovaries undergo cyclic alterations that may be associated with physiologically increased ^{18}F FDG uptake that is incidentally detected in patients with no known gynecologic malignancy. Moreover, adnexal and uterine lesions showing increased uptake are not always malignant. Benign lesions in these organs may show increased ^{18}F FDG uptake of variable intensity.[1,2]

Fusion of PET with computed tomography (CT) data can assist in localization of uptake as well as in defining the morphology of lesions, thus optimizing the diagnosis of the cause of increased tracer uptake in the pelvis.[2,3] In preparation for performing the PET/CT study, patients with gynecologic malignancies should be positioned for imaging with their hands above the head, whenever the patient can tolerate this position. Technical details are specifically related to imaging of the pelvis, including the known physiologic FDG activity in the bowel and urinary bladder, with its dynamic patterns on both PET and CT. Good hydration followed by complete voiding immediately before starting PET/CT acquisition are very important to reduce the high urinary tracer content as much as possible. Administration of diuretics or insertion of Foley catheters is seldom performed at present. The pelvis should be imaged at the beginning of the study to achieve a short time interval between the CT and PET components at this level, ensuring similar bladder size, volume, and shape.

This article summarizes the physiologic changes in the female reproductive system, which may be associated with increased ^{18}F FDG uptake, and the PET/CT appearance of adnexal and uterine benign lesions, which should be considered when reviewing PET/CT data of female patients with cancer.

Department of Nuclear Medicine, Tel Aviv Sourasky Medical Center, Sackler School of Medicine, Tel Aviv University, 6 Weizman Street, Tel Aviv, 64239 Israel
E-mail address: evensap@tasmc.health.gov.il

PET Clin 5 (2010) 425–434
doi:10.1016/j.cpet.2010.07.003
1556-8598/10/$ — see front matter © 2010 Elsevier Inc. All rights reserved.

PHYSIOLOGIC UPTAKE IN ENDOMETRIUM AND OVARIES

Physiologic Endometrial Uptake in Premenopausal Patients

The normal menstrual cycle reflects the fine balance between the proliferative action of estrogen and the secretory transforming action of progesterone on the endometrium. The menstrual cycle consists of 4 phases: menstrual flow, preovulatory, ovulatory, and secretory postovulation. Endometrial changes during the menstrual cycle involve proliferative and secretory changes and desquamation, because the abrupt reduction in estrogen and progesterone levels results in contraction of the coiled arteries supplying the endometrium, which is followed by ischemia and necrosis.[4,5]

Physiologic increased uptake of ^{18}F FDG in the endometrium in women in their reproductive age has 2 peaks; high-intensity uptake is present at the menstrual flow phase and low-intensity uptake at the ovulatory phase. Lerman and colleagues[6] have reported mean endometrial standard uptake values (SUVs) of 5 ± 3.2 in menstruating premenopausal patients, 3.7 ± 0.9 at the ovulatory phase, 2.6 ± 1.1 at the proliferative phase, and 2.5 ± 1.1 at the secretory phase. In a prospective study conducted by Nishizawa and colleagues[7] in healthy female volunteers, 78 were premenopausal, including 32 at the late follicular to early luteal phase showing increased endometrial uptake, with an SUV of 3.3 ± 0.3. In the first 3 days of the menstrual cycle, 9 women who were examined demonstrated intense uptake with an SUV of 4.6 ± 1.0.

Several hypotheses have been suggested to explain the cause of physiologic endometrial ^{18}F FDG uptake. Endometrial ^{18}F FDG uptake during menstruation may be related to the peristaltic movement of the subendometrial myometrium, which helps to discharge menstrual bleed.[8] There are 2 types of uterine movements: uterine peristalsis present during the ovulatory and menstrual phases and to a lesser extent in the luteal phase, which is a subtle movement limited to the subendometrial myometrium, and contractions of the subendometrial myometrium, which are stronger and observed particularly during menstruation and to a lesser extent at the periovulatory phase.[9-11] Kido and colleagues[8] evaluated the presence of a potential relationship between ^{18}F FDG uptake and uterine motility assessed by cine magnetic resonance (MR) imaging in 56 fertile women. Although there was no clear correlation between the peristaltic frequency and accumulation of ^{18}F FDG in the uterus, the latter was higher in patients with sustained contractions compared with patients with no contraction. Another possible cause for ^{18}F FDG uptake during menstruation is that this process exhibits some characteristics of inflammation. Leukocytes and cytokines emerge in the endometrium before the onset of menstruation, triggering tissue destruction. It has been postulated that these cytokines are induced by the sustained contractions observed in the luteal and menstrual phases, the menstrual cycle periods associated with increased endometrial ^{18}F FDG uptake.[12]

Assessing the activity of endometrial enzymes in 252 patients with normal menstruation cycles, Hughes[13] reported that the activity of glycogen synthetase causes increased synthesis of glycogen until midcycle followed by decreased levels of glycogen toward the end of the cycle, thus reflecting the role of glucose phosphorylation in the estrogenic stimulation of uterine glycolysis. Therefore, synthesis and breakdown of glycogen may be another cause for increased uptake of ^{18}F FDG in the endometrium.

Physiologic ^{18}F FDG uptake occurs in the endometrial region of the uterus, the cavity that is often but not always centrally located and can be identified on CT as a region of low attenuation. On sagittal views, physiologic endometrial uptake may be identified as a line of increased activity surrounded by the uterine walls that show no tracer uptake (**Fig. 1**). This pattern differs from uptake in a mass or due to increased mural activity, which often represent uterine malignancy or a benign myometrial pathologic condition, such as fibroids and polyps.[3,7] The position and shape of the uterus is significantly influenced by the degree of bladder distension.

Physiologic Ovarian Uptake in Premenopausal Patients

At each menstrual cycle during the reproductive age, a group of primordial follicles located at the ovarian cortex matures, with a single follicle becoming a preovulatory follicle. This follicle undergoes changes during the 7 days before ovulation. After that the postovulatory follicle is turned to a corpus luteum, which matures at the midluteal phase. In the corpus luteal cyst formed after ovulation, the follicular wall becomes vascularized, thickened, and partially collapsed.[14] The ovaries are oval-shaped structures located, as a rule, on both sides of the lesser pelvis close to the lateral wall. However, they may show a relatively large variability in location depending on their size, the degree of laxity of supporting ligaments, and previous pregnancies.

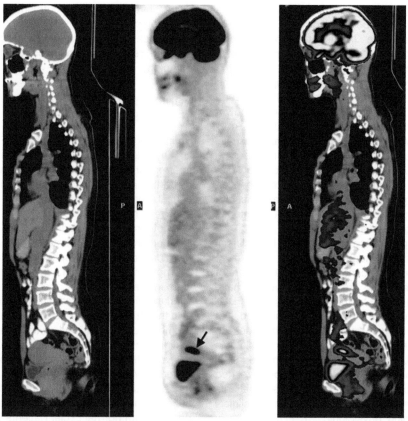

Fig. 1. Physiologic uptake of ^{18}F FDG during menstruation (sagittal images: CT [*left*], PET [*center*], PET/CT [*right*]). The centrally located increased linear tracer activity (*arrow*) is that of the endometrium. There is no increased tracer activity in the surrounding myometrium.

Potential causes for physiologic ^{18}F FDG uptake in the ovaries have been the scope of several earlier publications. It has been speculated that the ^{18}F FDG uptake in the ovaries reflects the enhanced Glut3 expression and increased glucose metabolism present in the ovaries in the preovulatory phase to meet the increased metabolic demands of the maturing follicle and the ovulated cumulus-enclosed oocyte.[15] Rupture of the follicle is considered to be an inflammatory reaction mediated by cytokines involving the presence of macrophages, which exhibit increased ^{18}F FDG accumulation.[16,17] The development of the corpus luteal cyst is a process somewhat similar to wound healing and tumor formation involving angiogenesis, which has also been related to increased accumulation of ^{18}F FDG.[17,18]

Lerman and colleagues[6] observed increased ^{18}F FDG uptake in the ovaries of 21 of 112 premenopausal patients without known gynecologic malignancy, including 15 patients at the time of ovulation with functional ovarian cysts detected on the CT component of PET/CT. Nishizawa and colleagues[7] reported increased ovarian uptake during the late follicular to early luteal phase in 26 of 78 premenopausal women. Physiologic uptake in the ovaries is temporary. Correlation between ovarian uptake and specific phases of the cycle was confirmed by Zhu and colleagues[19] who performed 4 to 6 follow-up studies on ^{18}F FDG-PET uptake at different menstruation phases in 14 premenopausal patients. In a study by Kim and colleagues,[20] increased ovarian uptake incidentally found in 15 female patients disappeared on a repeat short-term follow-up PET/CT. In this study, incidental ^{18}F FDG ovarian uptake was correlated with morphologic data obtained by MR imaging, CT, and ultrasonography (US). Ovarian uptake correlated in time to the late follicular, ovulatory, and early luteal to midluteal phases when the follicles and corpora lutea undergo active proliferation and not at the early follicular phase when follicles are small. The luteal phase is usually 14 ± 2 days in duration, whereas the length of the follicular phase varies between 1 to 3 weeks.[21] Physiologic ovarian uptake is therefore expected to occur between days 10 and 25 of the menstrual cycle. In the study by Kim and colleagues,[20] only 12 out of 38 premenopausal patients examined at days 10 to 25 of the menstrual cycle showed ovarian uptake. The investigators state that the reason for the absence of uptake in the remaining 26 patients is unknown.

Ovulatory follicle and corpus luteum may present as a focally increased uptake, usually unilateral, that is incidentally detected in the pelvis of premenopausal patients with no known ovarian malignancy. Follicular uptake appears spherical, and the corpus luteal uptake appears discoid. Usually, corpus luteal uptake is more intense than that of the ovulating follicle.[7]

The PET appearance of the ovaries is of clinical relevance in premenopausal patients who are at high risk for ovarian cancer, mainly the carriers of the BRCA gene who are already known to have breast malignancy. In these patients, ^{18}F FDG-PET/CT should be preferentially scheduled just after menstruation, thus reducing the need to debate whether the ovarian uptake is physiologic or abnormal. Ovarian uptake in premenopausal patients who had hysterectomy cannot be related to the menstruation cycle because these patients cannot report on their menstruation. In this clinical setting, defining physiologic ^{18}F FDG uptake in intact ovaries may occasionally require hormonal analysis.[22]

Postmenopausal Patients

In postmenopausal patients, neither the uterus nor the ovaries show intense increased physiologic uptake. Of 55 postmenopausal healthy volunteers, Nishizawa and colleagues[7] reported increased endometrial uptake in only 2 women with neglected intrauterine devices. Assessing 116 postmenopausal women with no known gynecologic malignancy, Lerman and colleagues[6] found the mean SUV of endometrial uptake to be lower than 1.6 in 111 patients. This uptake was measured by locating a region of interest at the center of the uterus where the endometrium is assumed to be present, because no significantly increased ^{18}F FDG uptake could be detected visually. This observation may reflect previous morphologic reports that showed that the postmenopausal endometrium is an active structure in a quiescent state rather than an atrophic state, mainly during the first few years of menopause.[23] Higher SUV of up to 4.5 was found in 5 postmenopausal patients in association with fibroid and polyps.[6]

Thus, because intense ^{18}F FDG uptake does not occur physiologically in postmenopausal women, detection of abnormal tracer activity in this patient group needs further assessment because it is likely to represent benign or malignant uterine pathology.

NONMALIGNANT ^{18}F FDG UPTAKE IN OVARIES AND UTERUS

Defining endometrial and ovarian ^{18}F FDG uptake as physiologic in patients with cancer who are referred for PET/CT imaging is not always possible by getting a menstrual history, because premenopausal oncologic patients may experience impaired menstruation cycle due to previous chemotherapy and radiotherapy. The risk of chemotherapy-related amenorrhea depends on the patient's age, specifically administered chemotherapeutic agent, and total dose. Older women have a higher incidence of complete ovarian failure and permanent infertility.[24]

In the study by Lerman and colleagues,[6] 24% of premenopausal patients with nongynecologic malignancies reported menstrual cycle irregularities after therapy. In patients with posttreatment oligomenorrhea, slightly increased endometrial and adnexal uptake was detected, similar to that seen in the ovulatory phase in premenopausal patients with normal cycle. Patients with amenorrhea resembled postmenopausal patients showing no physiologic increased uptake.

The use of oral contraceptives alters the endometrial and ovarian physiology.[25] Endometrial uptake in patients on birth control pills resembles that of nonovulating, nonmenstruating, premenopausal patients.[6]

The presence of an intrauterine device has been reported to be an occasional cause for constant ^{18}F FDG uptake secondary to associated inflammatory changes related to a foreign body reaction.[7] Recognizing the presence of this device on the CT component of the PET/CT study can be helpful in excluding a different cause for the increased tracer uptake.

Fertility preservation is considered before therapy in young female patients with cancer. The possibilities to preserve fertility include banking of mature oocytes or embryos after gonadotropin stimulation.[24,26] Therefore, hyperstimulated ovaries showing increased ^{18}F FDG uptake may be identified on a baseline PET/CT study before initiation of therapy (**Fig. 2**).

Antitumoral hormonal therapy with a nonsteroidal antiestrogen agent such as tamoxifen, prescribed for patients with breast cancer, has been associated with a high prevalence of

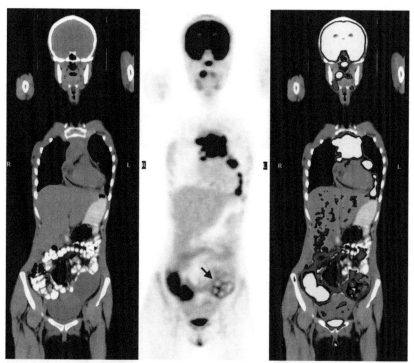

Fig. 2. Increased 18F FDG uptake (coronal images: CT [*left*], PET [*center*], PET/CT [*right*]) in multiple follicles within the left ovary (*arrow*) after gonadotropin stimulation for fertility preservation in a 26-year-old patient with newly diagnosed Hodgkin disease before therapy.

endometrial changes such as thickening, glandular hyperplasia, cystic atrophy, and formation of polyps and lesions, which may be associated with nontumoral endometrial low-intensity 18F FDG uptake.[6,27,28] Endometrial hyperplasia induced by tamoxifen can occur with or without cytologic atypia. In up to 23% of patients with atypical hyperplasia, hyperplasia progresses to carcinoma, whereas in only 2% of patients with hyperplasia without atypia hyperplasia progresses to carcinoma.[29] Therefore, increased 18F FDG uptake identified in a hyperplastic endometrium should be reported in these patients despite the high chances that it could be benign.

Young female patients with cervical, vaginal, or colorectal cancer in whom pelvic radiotherapy is considered undergo transposition of the ovaries outside the radiation field to preserve ovarian function. Transposed ovaries are usually positioned in the paracolic gutter or iliac fossa and maintain their physiologic characteristics. Therefore, the transposed ovaries can show physiologic increased 18F FDG uptake similar to intact ovaries in their original location but appear on PET/CT images as lower abdominal or high anterior pelvic masses. Misinterpretation of physiologic increased uptake in transposed ovaries as malignant implants may be avoided by obtaining a detailed history,

including previous surgical procedures. The presence of surgical clips next to the site of uptake on the CT component may hint the possibility of uptake in a transposed ovary (**Fig. 3**).[30,31]

Increased endometrial uptake, which is nonmalignant in nature, can be detected in patients with cervical cancer. The endometrium adjacent to the primary cervical tumor in premenopausal patients has been reported to show increased 18F FDG uptake with SUVs, similar to those measured during menstruation in premenopausal patients without gynecologic malignancy.[6,32] This increased 18F FDG uptake may be the result of stenosis caused by the primary cervical tumor with a consequent hydrometra (uterine fluid collection).[33] It is also possible that the local cytokine environment of the cervical tumor affects the adjacent endometrium, resulting in an altered 18F FDG uptake.[34] Contrast-enhanced MR imaging is considered to be the accurate imaging modality for determining the local extent of disease.[35]

18F FDG UPTAKE IN BENIGN LESIONS IN THE OVARIES AND UTERUS

In addition to malignant tumors, benign ovarian and uterine lesions may accumulate 18F FDG.[36] Benign FDG-avid lesions of the ovaries include

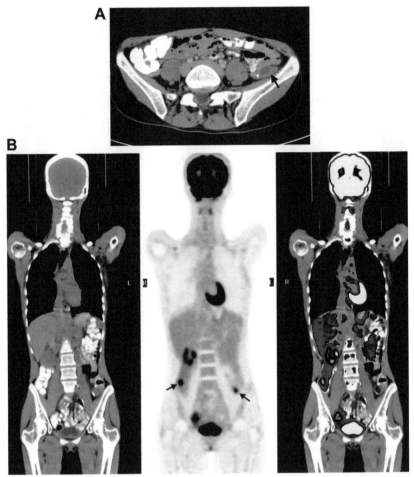

Fig. 3. Increased ^{18}F FDG uptake in transposed ovaries. (*A*) Transaxial CT image demonstrates the presence of a transposed ovary with follicle at the left gutter, anterior to a surgical clip (*arrow*). Similar findings were detected on CT on the right gutter (not shown). (*B*) Increased physiologic ^{18}F FDG uptake (coronal images: CT [*left*], PET [*center*], PET/CT [*right*]) in both the transposed ovaries (*arrows*).

follicular ovarian cysts and hemorrhagic luteus, among other causes. Frenchel and colleagues[37] compared PET findings in 99 patients with asymptomatic adnexal masses with that of histopathology, transvaginal B-mode and Doppler US, and MR imaging. Overlapping intensity of ^{18}F FDG uptake was found in tumors of low malignant potential, early-stage ovarian carcinomas, and benign adnexal lesions. Rieber and colleagues[38] evaluated the diagnostic performance of MR imaging, transvaginal sonography, and ^{18}F FDG-PET in 103 patients with asymptomatic adnexal findings. Increased ^{18}F FDG uptake was found in 19 of 91 cases of benign ovarian processes, including cystadenoma, endometrioma, hydrosalpinx, benign germ cell tumors, cholesterol granuloma, abscess, and thecoma, and in 4 of 22 endometriomas diagnosed in this study. It therefore seems that ^{18}F FDG uptake cannot differentiate between malignant and benign adnexal lesions.

In sporadic cases, increased ^{18}F FDG uptake has been described in relation with endometriosis.[39] This entity is defined by the presence of endometrial-like glandular epithelium and stroma in ectopic locations. The ovaries are the most frequent anatomic location for endometriosis, but other locations, such as pelvic and extrapelvic, have also been observed. In general, endometrial implants behave like the normal endometrium in their response to hormones, with estrogen stimulating growth and progesterone inhibiting growth. However, most endometrial implants do not have the cyclic histologic changes characteristic of normal endometrium.[40,41] It is therefore possible that the cause of ^{18}F FDG uptake in endometriosis is not necessarily related to cyclic endometrial changes but is the result of inflammation.

Activated macrophages and inflammatory cells, frequently present in endometriotic lesions, can cause increased tracer uptake.[39] The role of 18F FDG-PET in imaging endometriosis is yet to be explored.

Increased 18F FDG uptake has been described in uterine leiomyomas, endometrial hyperplasia and polyps, and pyometra (**Fig. 4**).[3] Up to 18% of benign fibroid uterine tumors can be FDG-avid. Leiomyomas are the most common human uterine neoplasm, composed of smooth muscle with varying amounts of fibrous connective tissue and occur in over 25% of women aged 35 years and older.[42,43] Most leiomyomas show only minimal or mild 18F FDG uptake, with intense tracer activity being described in some cases. However, the detection of high-intensity 18F FDG uptake in leiomyomas needs further investigation to exclude the presence of leiomyosarcomas because in rare cases, less than 1% of leiomyomas may undergo malignant degeneration.[44] Neither the pathophysiology of uterine leiomyomas nor the cause for 18F FDG uptake in these benign lesions is fully understood. It is known that steroid sex hormones, mainly progesterone, play an important role in the regulation of the growth of leiomyoma.[42,45] Increased vascularity, high levels of growth factors and receptors related to proliferation of smooth muscle, and high levels of granulocyte-macrophage colony-stimulating factors also play a role in the pathophysiology of leiomyomas. The normal and myomatous uteruses

differ in their expression of basic fibroblast growth factor (bFGF) and its receptors, with the myomatous uterus having higher levels of bFGF. The bFGF is an angiogenic growth factor that promotes the formation of new blood vessels and causes proliferation of smooth muscle cells. Leiomyoma tissue exhibits significantly higher levels of epidermal growth factor (EGF) messenger RNA than the normal myometrium. It has been postulated that both estradiol and progesterone coordinate their effects on EGF by upregulating its receptors and EGF-like proteins.[42,44] These factors are probably responsible for the uptake of 18F FDG in leiomyomas. Also, this hormonal dependency of uptake seems to be supported by a lower incidence of 18F FDG uptake in leiomyomas in postmenopausal compared with premenopausal women.[42,46] Nishizawa and colleagues[47] reviewed 18F FDG-PET and pelvic MR images of 477 premenopausal and 880 postmenopausal women with no known gynecologic diseases. Leiomyomas were found in 164 premenopausal and 338 postmenopausal women. 18F FDG uptake was observed in 10.4% of leiomyomas in premenopausal women and in only 1.2% of leiomyomas in postmenopausal women. However, 18F FDG uptake in leiomyomas is not explained solely by the effect of hormones.[43] By correlating scintigraphic findings with MR images, it was found that most leiomyomas that do not demonstrate increased 18F FDG uptake have low signal intensity on T2-weighted MR imaging, whereas lesions

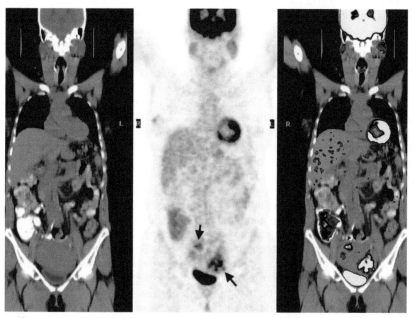

Fig. 4. Increased 18F FDG uptake (coronal images: CT [*left*], PET [*center*], PET/CT [*right*]) in benign uterine leiomyomas (*arrows*).

that accumulate ^{18}F FDG show signal intensity equal to or higher than that of the myometrium, which suggests a correlation between cellularity and uptake. Of note, an earlier publication reported that cellularity-influenced ^{18}F FDG uptake only in the presence of GLUT-1, the positive expression of which provides a potential explanation on why not all leiomyomas with increased signal intensity on T2-weighted MR images show increased ^{18}F FDG uptake.[48]

To assess the relationship between age, size, degree of degeneration, and contrast enhancement on MR imaging and ^{18}F FDG uptake in leiomyomas, Kitajima and colleagues[46] investigated 61 lesions in 41 patients who underwent PET/CT and contrast-enhanced MR imaging. Leiomyomas were divided into nondegenerated lesions showing low and intermediate signal intensity on T2- and T1-weighted images, respectively, and degenerated leiomyomas showing other types of signal intensity. Leiomyomas were also divided into strongly and weakly enhancing lesions based on the degree of contrast enhancement on MR imaging. There was a moderate negative correlation between the ^{18}F FDG measured SUVs and age and a mild positive correlation between SUVs and size. Maximum SUV of degenerated lesions was higher than that of nondegenerated leiomyomas. These findings suggest that heterogeneity in cellularity, degeneration, and the degree of proliferation of leiomyomas can explain the differences in their metabolic demand and subsequently in the degree of ^{18}F FDG uptake in general as well as in the focal uptake in different regions of a single leiomyoma, mainly in large lesions.

SUMMARY

Increased ^{18}F FDG uptake in the uterus and ovaries may be physiologic in premenopausal patients. In young women with a normal menstruation cycle, knowledge of the menstrual history and characteristic patterns of physiologic ^{18}F FDG uptake on PET/CT may assist in avoiding false-positive interpretations. It is also important to obtain the patient's history regarding the use of contraceptives, ovarian hyperstimulation for fertility preservation, previous ovarian transposition surgery, and treatment with antitumoral hormonal therapy. Intense ^{18}F FDG uptake in the ovaries and uterus in postmenopausal patients with unknown gynecologic cancer required further investigation because it is often associated with benign or malignant pathology. [18]F FDG-PET/CT cannot differentiate between benign and malignant lesions with a high degree of certainty because both may show ^{18}F FDG uptake of overlapping intensity in the ovaries and uterus.

REFERENCES

1. Cook GJR, Fogelman I, Maisey MN. Normal physiological and benign pathological variants of 18-fluoro-2-deoxyglucose positron-emission tomography scanning: potential for error in interpretation. Semin Nucl Med 1996;26:308–14.
2. Subhas N, Patel PV, Pannu HK, et al. Imaging of pelvic malignancies with in-line FDG PET-CT: case examples and common pitfalls of FDG PET. Radiographics 2005;25:1031–43.
3. Liu Y. Benign ovarian and endometrial uptake on FDG PET-CT: patterns and pitfalls. Ann Nucl Med 2009;23:107–12.
4. Rebar RW. The normal menstrual cycle. In: Keye WR, editor. Infertility: evaluation and treatment. Philadelphia: Saunders; 1995. p. 85.
5. Hale GE, Hughes CL, Cline JM. Endometrial cancer: hormonal factors, the perimenopausal "window of risk," and isoflavones. J Clin Endocrinol Metab 2002;87:3–15.
6. Lerman H, Metser U, Grisaru D, et al. Normal and abnormal 18F-FDG endometrial and ovarian uptake in pre- and postmenopausal patients: assessment by PET/CT. J Nucl Med 2004;45:266–71.
7. Nishizawa S, Inubushi M, Okada H. Physiological 18F-FDG uptake in the ovaries and uterus of healthy female volunteers. Eur J Nucl Med Mol Imaging 2005;32:549–56.
8. Kido A, Nakamoto Y, Nishizawa S, et al. Physiological uptake of 18F-fluorodeoxyglucose in uterine endometrium and myometrium: correlation with uterine motility evaluated by cine magnetic resonance imaging. Acta Radiol 2009;50:455–61.
9. Kunz G, Leyendecker G. Uterine peristaltic activity during the menstrual cycle: characterization, regulation, function and dysfunction. Reprod Biomed Online 2002;4(Suppl 2):5–9.
10. Nakai A, Togashi K, Yamaoka T, et al. Uterine peristalsis shown on cine MR imaging using ultrafast sequence. J Magn Reson Imaging 2003;18:726–33.
11. Fujiwara T, Togashi K, Yamaoka T, et al. Kinematics of the uterus: cine mode MR imaging. Radiographics 2004;24:e19.
12. Kelly RW, Illingworth P, Baldie G, et al. Progesterone control of interleukin-8 production in endometrium and chorio-decidual cells underlines the role of the neutrophil in menstruation and parturition. Hum Reprod 1994;9:253–8.
13. Hughes EC. The effect of enzymes upon metabolism, storage, and release of carbohydrates in normal and abnormal endometria. Cancer 1976;38:487–502.

14. Borders R, Breiman RS, Yeh BM, et al. Computed tomography of corpus luteal cysts. J Comput Assist Tomogr 2004;28:340–2.

15. Kol S, Ben-Shlomo I, Ruutiainen K, et al. The mid-cycle increase in ovarian glucose uptake is associated with enhanced expression of glucose transporter 3. J Clin Invest 1997;99:2274–83.

16. Kubota R, Yamada S, Kubota K, et al. Intratumoral distribution of fluorine-18-fluorodeoxyglucose in vivo: high accumulation in macrophages and granulation tissues studied by microautoradiography. J Nucl Med 1992;33:1972–80.

17. Vanatier D, Dufour P, Tordjeman-Rizzi N, et al. Immunological aspects of ovarian function: role of the cytokines. Eur J Obstet Gynecol Reprod Biol 1995; 63:155–68.

18. Smith MF, McIntush EW, Smith GW. Mechanism associated with corpus luteum development. J Anim Sci 1994;72:1857–72.

19. Zhu Z, Wang B, Cheng W, et al. Endometrial and ovarian 18F-FDG uptake in serial PET studies and the value of delayed imaging for differentiation. Clin Nucl Med 2006;31:781–7.

20. Kim SK, Kang KW, Roh JW, et al. Incidental ovarian 18F-FDG accumulation on PET: correlation with the menstrual cycle. Eur J Nucl Med Mol Imaging 2005;32:757–63.

21. Balsara G, Hernandez E. The ovary: normal, physiologic changes, endometriosis, and metastatic tumors. In: Hernandez E, Atkinson BF, editors. Clinical gynecologic pathology. Philadelphia: Saunders; 1995. p. 404–9.

22. Nishizawa S, Inubushi M, Ozawa F, et al. Physiological FDG uptake in the ovaries after hysterectomy. Ann Nucl Med 2007;21:345–8.

23. Noci I, Borri P, Scarselli G, et al. Morphological and functional aspects of the endometrium of asymptomatic post-menopausal women: does the endometrium really age? Hum Reprod 1996;11:2246–50.

24. Maltaris T, Beckmann MW, Dittrich R. Fertility preservation for young female cancer patients. In Vivo 2009;23:123–30.

25. Lobo RA, Stanczyk FZ. New knowledge in the physiology of hormonal contraceptives. Am J Obstet Gynecol 1994;170:1499–507.

26. Blumenfeld Z. How to preserve fertility in young women exposed to chemotherapy? The role of GnRH agonist cotreatment in addition to cryopreservation of embryo, oocytes, or ovaries. Oncologist 2007;12:1044–54.

27. Levine D, Gosink B, Johnson LA. Change in endometrial thickness in postmenopausal women undergoing hormone replacement therapy. Radiology 1995;197:603–8.

28. Ascher MS, Imaoka I, Lang MJ. Tamoxifen-induced uterine abnormalities: the role of imaging. Radiology 2000;214:29–38.

29. Kurman RJ, Norris HJ. Endometrial hyperplasia and related cellular changes. In: Kurman RJ, editor. Blaustein's pathology of the female genital tract. 4th edition. New York: Springer-Verlag; 1994. p. 411–43.

30. Zissin R, Metser U, Lerman H, et al. PET-CT findings in surgically transposed ovaries. Br J Radiol 2006; 79:110–5.

31. Chung HH, Kang WJ, Kim JW, et al. Characterization of surgically transposed ovaries in integrated PET/CT in patients with cervical cancer. Acta Obstet Gynecol Scand 2007;86:88–93.

32. Tsujikawa T, Yoshida Y, Mori T, et al. Uterine tumors: pathophysiologic imaging with 16alpha-[18F]fluoro-17beta-estradiol and 18F fluorodeoxyglucose PET—initial experience. Radiology 2008;248: 599–605.

33. Breckenridge JW, Kurtz AB, Ritchie WGM, et al. Postmenopausal uterine fluid collection: indicator of carcinoma. AJR Am J Roentgenol 1982;139: 529–34.

34. Imai A, Matsunami K, Ohno T, et al. Enhancement of growth-promoting activity in extract from uterine cancers by protein kinase C in human endometrial fibroblasts. Gynecol Obstet Invest 1992;33:109–13.

35. Sahdev A, Reznek RH. Magnetic resonance imaging of endometrial and cervical cancer. Ann N Y Acad Sci 2008;1138:214–32.

36. Castellucci P, Perrone AM, Picchio M, et al. Diagnostic accuracy of 18F-FDG PET-CT in characterizing ovarian lesions and staging ovarian cancer: correlation with transvaginal ultrasound, computed tomography and history. Nucl Med Commun 2007; 28:589–95.

37. Frenchel S, Grab D, Nuessle K, et al. Asymptomatic adnexal masses: correlation of FDG PET and histopathologic findings. Radiology 2002;223:780–8.

38. Rieber A, Nussle K, Stohr I, et al. Preoperative diagnosis of ovarian tumors with MR imaging: comparison with transvaginal sonography, positron emission tomography and histologic findings. AJR Am J Roentgenol 2001;177:123–9.

39. Jeffry L, Kerrou K, Camatte S, et al. Endometriosis with FDG uptake on PET. Eur J Obstet Gynecol Reprod Biol 2004;117:236–9.

40. Van Gorp T, Amant F, Neven P, et al. Endometriosis and the development of malignant tumors of the pelvis. A review of literature. Best Pract Res Clin Obstet Gynaecol 2004;18:349–71.

41. Olive DL, Schwartz LB. Endometriosis. N Engl J Med 1993;328:1759–69.

42. Houston KD, Hunter DS, Hodges LC, et al. Uterine leiomyomas: mechanisms of tumorigenesis. Toxicol Pathol 2001;29:100–4.

43. Lin CY, Ding HJ, Chen YK, et al. F-18 FDG PET in detecting uterine leiomyoma. Clin Imaging 2008;32: 38–41.

44. Blake RE. Lelomyomata uteri: hormonal and molecular determinants of growth. J Natl Med Assoc 2007;99:1170–84.

45. Chura JC, Truskinovsky AM, Judson PL, et al. Positron emission tomography and leiomyomas: clinicopathologic analysis of 3 cases of PET scan positive leiomyomas and literature review. Gynecol Oncol 2007;104:247–52.

46. Kitajima K, Murakami K, Yamasaki E, et al. Standardized uptake values of uterine leiomyoma with 18F-FDG PET/CT: variation with age, size, degeneration, and contrast enhancement on MRI. Ann Nucl Med 2008;22:505–12.

47. Nishizawa S, Inubushi M, Kido A, et al. Incidence and characteristics of uterine leiomyomas with FDG uptake. Ann Nucl Med 2008;22:803–10.

48. Higashi T, Tamaki N, Torizuka T, et al. FDG uptake, GLUT-1 glucose transporter and cellularity in human pancreatic tumors. J Nucl Med 1998;39: 1727–35.

The Role of FDG-PET/CT in Cervical Cancer: Diagnosis, Staging, Radiation Treatment Planning and Follow-Up

Elesyia D. Haynes-Outlaw, MD[a], Perry W. Grigsby, MD[b,c],*

KEYWORDS

- Cervical cancer • Radiotherapy treatment planning
- PET • Cancer staging

The advent of routine Papanicolaou (Pap) smears has lead to a substantial reduction in the incidence and greater than 70% decrease in mortality of cervical cancer over the last 50 years.[1] This screening tool can detect abnormalities in the cervical epithelial cells before clinically apparent tumors arise. The American Cancer Society Facts and Figures estimated 11,270 new cases of cervical cancer and 4070 deaths in the United States for 2009.[2] Despite this progress in the West, cervical cancer continues to represent a significant problem in developing countries. An estimated 500,000 women are diagnosed yearly with more than 250,000 deaths in recent years.[3]

Several prospective randomized trials of chemoradiation compared with radiation alone for advanced cervical cancer showed substantial improvement in local control and overall survival.[4–8] As a result, the National Cancer Institute issued a treatment alert in 1999 establishing chemoradiation as the standard of care in these patients. Despite chemoradiation, approximately one-third of patients with advanced cervical cancer will have disease recurrence and most will also have evidence of local failure.[4]

Even within developed countries, there are disparate resources and debates regarding the optimal workup and management of patients with cervical cancer. The International Federation of Gynecologists & Obstetricians (FIGO) continues to be the most widely accepted staging system for cervical cancer. However, there is mounting evidence suggesting that the additional use of imaging modalities, both anatomic-based, such as CT and MR imaging, as well as metabolic imaging tests, such as PET, may provide important diagnostic and prognostic information.[9–11] This review summarizes the salient papers on the use of PET and hybrid PET/CT imaging using the glucose analog ^{18}F-fluoro-2-deoxy-D-glucose

This work was supported by Grant 5 KL2 RRO24983-03 from the National Center for Research Resources, a component of the National Institutes of Health.
Conflict of interest: The authors have no conflict of interest to disclose.
[a] Department of Radiation Oncology, University of Texas Southwestern Medical Center, MC 9183, Dallas, Texas 75390-9183, USA
[b] Nuclear Medicine and Gynecologic Oncology, Washington University School of Medicine, 4921 Parkview Place, St Louis, MO 63110, USA
[c] Brachytherapy & MicroRT Treatment Center, Mallinckrodt Institute of Radiology, Washington University School of Medicine, 4921 Parkview Place, St Louis, MO 63110, USA
* Corresponding author. Department of Radiation Oncology, Washington University School of Medicine, Box 8224, St Louis, Missouri 63110.
E-mail address: pgrigsby@wustl.edu

PET Clin 5 (2010) 435–446
doi:10.1016/j.cpet.2010.07.004

(FDG) in the diagnosis, staging, radiation treatment planning, and follow-up of cervical cancers.

DIAGNOSIS

In the vast majority of patients, cervical cancer usually develops through a well-characterized pattern of cytologic changes in the epithelium caused by human papillomavirus. Preinvasive changes, such as atypical squamous cells of uncertain significance, low-grade squamous intraepithelial lesion, or cervical intraepithelial neoplasia, then progress to high-grade squamous intraepithelial neoplasia, cervical intraepithelial neoplasia, or carcinoma in situ. Diagnosis of these preinvasive states as well as of early stage cervical cancer before the development of visible tumors or symptoms is made, as a rule, by Pap testing or colposcopy. Early detection of cervical cancer portends a survival advantage and therefore routine screening for cervical cancer is recommended for women aged 21 to 70 years.[3]

Patients with advanced or symptomatic cervical cancers usually have clinically apparent tumors with the final diagnosis being made via direct biopsy. Symptoms usually follow a predictable pattern progressing from postcoital bleeding to metrorrhagia or menorrhagia and foul smelling discharge, associated at a later stage with chronic anemia, and rectal or bladder symptoms in patients with advanced tumors.[3] Squamous cell carcinomas account for the overwhelming majority (>90%) of cervical cancers with adenocarcinoma and tumors of other histology, such as clear cell, small cell, or adenosquamous, making up the remaining cases. An initial cervical mass can be also occasionally found during workup for other gastrointestinal or genitourinary complaints. Because cervical cancer is usually detected by Pap test or clinical examination, there is only limited data on the use of imaging modalities including FDG-PET/CT in the primary detection of these malignancies.

STAGING

As mentioned previously, staging of cervical cancer is done in accordance with the FIGO clinical criteria, which allows information obtained from physical examination, including examination under anesthesia, lesion biopsy, endocervical curettage, hysteroscopy, cystoscopy, proctoscopy, barium enema, intravenous pyelogram (IVP), and radiographs of the chest and skeleton, to be used for staging purposes. This criteria allows uniform staging evaluation of patients with

cervical cancer worldwide and facilitates treatment outcome comparison.[1]

Surgical correlation studies have shown that physical examination has a limited ability to approximate the true size and extent of the tumor when compared with pathologic specimens.[12–15] Discrepancies between clinical and surgical staging range from about 25% in early stage disease (≤Stage IIA) to 65% to 90% in more advanced tumors (≥Stage IIB).[16] FIGO-allowed evaluation provides a paucity of information on lymph node status, which can, however, have a substantial impact on planning the treatment strategy in patients with presumed early stage tumors.[17] Cervical cancer spreads in a predictable pattern from the primary tumor to pelvic, para-aortic, supraclavicular lymph nodes and then to non-nodal distant sites. It is rare to have extrapelvic disease without pelvic lymph node involvement.[3,18,19]

Although data obtained from other modalities will not affect the FIGO clinical staging, it provides important information that may affect further management. Modalities, such as lymphangiography and surgical staging, have fallen out of routine use, although surgical staging is still advocated as the gold standard to assess pelvic and para-aortic lymph node metastasis.[20] Prior to the advent of metabolic imaging, anatomic-based radiologic techniques, such as CT and MR imaging, were the noninvasive modalities of choice to assess locoregional involvement. CT provided an important innovation in the work-up of cervical cancers in the pre-MR imaging era.[21–23] CT can simultaneously assess regional lymph nodes and the presence of hydronephrosis with relative ease as compared with historical methods, such as lymphangiography and intravenous pyelography (IVP).

However, CT has a limited ability to differentiate between tumor and adjacent normal tissue in the cervix or parametrium, with a sensitivity estimate of 55%.[16] Tumor invasion into the cervical stroma and early parametrium invasion was studied using CT, MR imaging and PET. CT can understage the pelvic sidewall involvement in patients with advanced disease.[24] MR imaging has been shown to be of value in imaging the primary lesion in cervical cancers. In a seminal study, Hricak and Phillips[24] evaluated 57 consecutive subjects with cervical cancer who had undergone surgical resection and showed that MR imaging had accuracies for detecting parametrial, pelvic sidewall, bladder, and rectal involvement of 88%, 95%, 96%, and 100%, respectively. The overall staging accuracy was 88%.[25] A good correlation (r = 0.98) was found between 3-dimensional (3-D) MR imaging volumetric analysis and 3-D tumor measurements on surgical specimens.[26-28] Subsequently, Mayr and colleagues[29] conducted a prospective study evaluating 3-D MR imaging and physical examination in 43 subjects with advanced cervical cancer before the start of therapy, after administration of radiotherapy at a dose of 20 to 25 Gy, at 45 to 50 Gy, and 1 to 2 months posttreatment. Results of this study showed suboptimal correlation between physical examination and 3-D MR imaging, r = 0.58. A prospective study comparing clinical examination, CT and MR imaging in assessing pelvic tumor volume in subjects with cervical cancer demonstrated the superiority of MR imaging in evaluating tumor size and uterine body involvement.[9] Based on these data MR imaging is being recommended as the gold standard for noninvasive evaluation of tumor size and extension of cervical cancer.[20]

Several studies have been published evaluating the efficacy of CT and MR imaging to assess lymph node involvement in cervical cancer.[30-38] Despite their prime spatial resolution, both CT and MR imaging are suboptimal for evaluation of nodal disease.[11,16,39,40] These techniques rely on size to define the presence of metastatic lymphadenopathy and nodes with a short-axis diameter of greater than 1 cm are generally thought to be involved with disease.[11] This criterion has multiple drawbacks, including the fact that it can miss and leave undetected metastases in lymph nodes smaller than 1cm and also that there are multiple nonmalignant causes for the presence of enlarged lymph nodes. These drawbacks limit the utility of CT and MR imaging for regional lymph node staging with estimated sensitivities of 43% and 60%, respectively in one meta-analysis.[16]

FDG-PET and PET/CT Staging of Cervical Cancer

PET is a functional imaging modality that, using FDG, provides information about regional glucose metabolism. Because FDG-PET relies on increased glucose uptake and metabolism within tumors compared with the surrounding normal tissue, it has a distinct advantage by not solely depending on anatomy. Physiologic changes usually precede structural alterations,[10] which has allowed FDG-PET to become a well-established tool in the primary evaluation of multiple malignancies.[41-46]

Primary Site Evaluation

Multiple studies have investigated the value of FDG-PET in assessing primary cervical cancer.[47-51] A study by Miller and Grigsby[52] described a 3-D quantitative technique measuring primary cervical cancer tumor volume. The 40% threshold value of the standard uptake value of maximal glucose uptake (SUV_{max}) within the tumor demonstrated a high correlation with CT and MR imaging, r = 0.88. A recent report by Showalter and colleagues[49] assessed the relationship between preoperative FDG-PET measured and pathologic tumor size in a prospective cohort of 40 subjects with early stage cervical cancer undergoing radical hysterectomy. This study demonstrated an excellent coefficient of determination, R^2 = 0.95, between the FDG-PET and surgical specimen measurements. The same good results have also been reported in larger tumors.[47,53]

Historical prognostic factors, such as tumor stage, size and histology, patient age, and lymph node status, have been well documented for cervical cancer.[20,54] The aforementioned study by Miller and Grigsby[52] showed improved overall survival in subjects with tumor volume less than 60 cm^3 compared with larger tumors, P = .003. In addition to primary tumor volume delineation, FDG-PET also provides important prognostic information regarding the patient response to chemoradiation, pelvic recurrence, and survival.[52,55] Measurement of pretreatment SUV_{max} in the primary tumor identified 3 prognostic groups; based on values of less than or equal to 5.2, 5.2 to 13.3, and greater than 13.3, subjects with cervical cancer had 5-year overall survival rates of 95%, 70%, and 44%, respectively. SUV_{max} was not clearly associated with clinical stage or tumor volume but was predictive of lymph node involvement, P = .0009.[55] A prognostic value of SUVmax measurements has also been reported for other malignancies, such as lung and head and neck cancers.[56-61]

Regional Lymph Node Evaluation

FDG-PET has a superior ability to detect regional and distant metastatic disease in patients with cervical cancer as compared with CT and MR imaging (Fig. 1).[10,40,47,62-64] In a retrospective analysis of 59 subjects with Stage IA-IIA disease, Wright and colleagues[65] reported that FDG-PET before definitive surgery had a sensitivity and specificity of 53% and 90% respectively for detection of metastases. Combining preoperative contrast-enhanced CT with FDG-PET findings in 42 of these subjects led to an increase in sensitivity to 75%.

Other authors have assessed the role of FDG-PET in locally advanced cervical cancer.[47,53] One of the earliest studies was published by Rose and colleagues[47] who performed FDG-PET before surgical staging in 32 subjects with stage IIB-IVA disease. FDG-PET had a sensitivity of 75% and

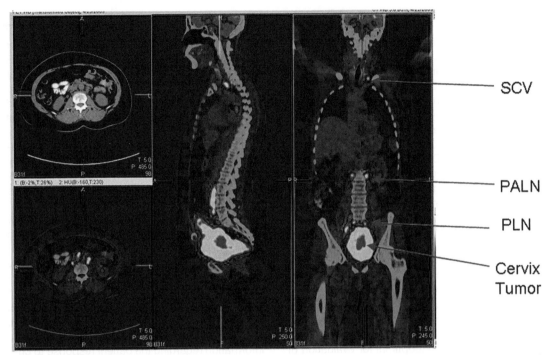

Fig. 1. Staging PET/CT study showing a large primary cervical cancer with an occult left supraclavicular metastasis (*red arrows*).

specificity of 92% in detecting para-aortic lymph node metastases and a sensitivity of 100% and specificity of 100% in 17 subjects who underwent pelvic node lymphadenectomy. Additionally, Singh and colleagues[53] evaluated 47 subjects with stage IIIB disease who underwent pretreatment FDG-PET. In 28% of the subjects FDG-PET did not demonstrate nodal involvement, 43% had positive pelvic nodes, 15% had pelvic and para-aortic nodal involvement, and 15% of the subjects had positive pelvic, para-aortic, and supraclavicular nodes. The 3-year cause-specific survival in each of these groups was of 73%, 58%, 29%, and 0%, respectively ($P = .0005$). In a separate analysis, Tran and colleagues[66] evaluated 14 subjects with newly diagnosed cervical cancer who had occult left supraclavicular metastases on baseline FDG-PET. These subjects underwent ultrasound-guided fine-needle aspiration to the specific FDG-positive sites, with metastatic disease further confirmed in all 14 subjects. This finding resulted in a positive predictive value (PPV) of 100% in supraclavicular lymph nodes and to further poor outcome in this subject subset. More recently, SUV_{max} measurements in involved lymph nodes suggest that this semiquantitative index should be used as a significant prognostic biomarker in patients with newly diagnosed advanced cervical cancer.[56,67]

FDG-PET/CT FOR TREATMENT PLANNING
Conventional Radiation Therapy

One of the most exciting areas for the use of FDG-PET in cervical cancer is radiation treatment planning. Traditionally, conventional external beam radiation therapy for cervical cancer consisted of a 4-field whole pelvic radiation. As previously mentioned, the advent of metabolic imaging has facilitated a more accurate detection of metastatic para-aortic lymph nodes. This accuracy has further allowed modifying radiation portals to incorporate involved lymph nodes via additional anterior posterior - posterior anterior fields. The dose delivered to disease-bearing sites was limited by small-bowel tolerance for whole pelvic fields. For para-aortic fields, specifically spinal cord and kidney, doses also had to be considered.

Intensity Modulated Radiation Therapy

As the ability to identify and subsequently target locoregional disease in cervical cancer has increased, more advanced radiation therapy techniques, such as intensity modulated radiation therapy (IMRT) and subsequently FDG-PET/CT image-guided IMRT, have been investigated. IMRT allows defining radiation fields that can spare or decrease the dose to adjacent normal tissues. This technique is of similar utility in treatment planning of head and neck and prostate cancer.[68,69] The feasibility of IMRT for small-bowel sparing in gynecologic cancer has been reported by multiple investigators.[70–74]

Roeske and colleagues[70] compared the administration of 45 Gy via conventional whole pelvic radiation to 9-field IMRT pelvic radiation. The IMRT plan reduced the volume of small bowel receiving the prescription dose from 33.8% to 17.4% ($P = .0005$). IMRT planning has also significantly reduced the volume of the rectum and urinary bladder receiving 45 Gy. The incidence and intensity of acute toxicity in patients with gynecologic malignancies following IMRT has been compared with conventional whole pelvic radiation. IMRT led to significantly less grade 2 gastrointestinal (GI) toxicity ($P = .002$), less use of antidiarrheal medication ($P = .001$), and less grade 2 genitourinary toxicity (10% vs 20%, although not statistically significant).[71,72] Two studies have demonstrated that IMRT with extended fields for treatment of para-aortic lymph nodes is feasible.[73,74]

Macdonald and colleagues[75] have prospectively assessed the value of a pseudo-step wedge (PSW) technique using FDG-PET/CT image-guided IMRT. Although 45 Gy to the whole pelvis along with brachytherapy is routinely given, the Mallinckrodt Institute of Radiology has a long history of using a central block after 20 Gy.[3] The rationale behind this technique is to shield the bladder and rectum and thus to decrease toxicity while giving higher doses with brachytherapy aiming to improve local control. The study was designed to replicate this dose distribution with IMRT. All subjects underwent FDG-PET/CT simulation in treatment position. The primary tumor in the cervix was defined on the fused FDG-PET/CT images as the metabolic tumor volume (MTV$_{cervix}$). The pelvic vessels were contoured from the aortic bifurcation to the level of the midfemoral heads and a 2 cm margin, excluding pelvic bones, femoral heads, and vertebral bodies, was used to create the nodal clinical target volume (CTV$_{nodal}$). A 0.7 cm margin was added to create the planning target volume (PTV$_{final}$ [**Figs. 2** and **3**]). Several organs at risk were contoured for each plan, including the skin, bladder, rectum, kidneys, femurs, pelvic bones, vertebral bodies, spinal cord, and bowel (both the small and large intestines). The treatment aimed to deliver 50.4 Gy to the PTV$_{final}$ and 20.0 Gy to MTV$_{cervix}$ along with brachytherapy cervix boost. This dose was considered as equivalent to a 85 Gy low dose rate equivalent to Point A. These plans were compared with 4-field conventional radiation to

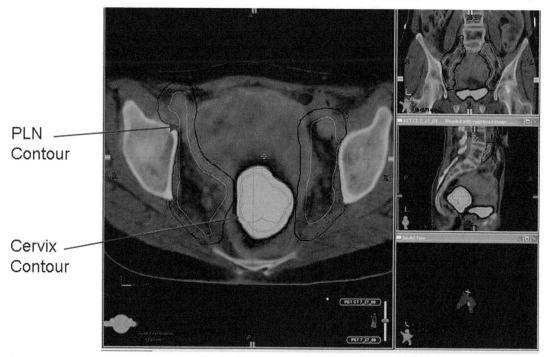

PLN Contour

Cervix Contour

Fig. 2. PET/CT for treatment planning showing the metabolic tumor volume in the cervix (MTVcervix, *green line* and *lower arrow*). The contours for pelvic vessels and CTVnodal for the pelvic lymph nodes are shown in yellow and red (*upper arrow*), respectively.

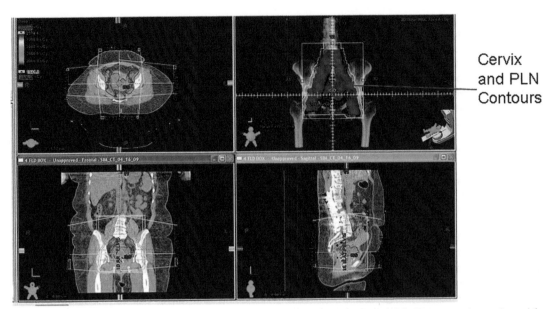

Cervix
and PLN
Contours

Fig. 3. Standard 4 field pelvic fields with MTVcervix cervical tumor and CTVnodal (*magenta, red arrow*) used for image-guided IMRT treatment planning.

45 Gy and whole pelvic IMRT to 45 Gy, both also with brachytherapy cervix boost. Dose volume histogram (DVH) analysis demonstrated that the PSW technique delivered significantly higher doses to Points A and P, similar doses to the rectal point, and was responsible for a significantly higher bladder point dose compared with the other techniques. Outcome assessed on the 3-month post-treatment FDG-PET/CT was consistent with previous institutional data and the acute toxicity was acceptable. Based on these results this technique has become, with minor modifications, the standard practice for patients with intact cervical cancer at the authors' institution.[75]

Esthappan and colleagues[76] outlined a treatment technique using FDG-PET/CT image-guided IMRT for dose escalation with positive para-aortic lymph nodes in a prospective clinical trial.[77] All subjects underwent PET/CT simulation in the treatment position. The pelvic and para-aortic regions were contoured from the renal vessels to the medial circumflex artery plus a 0.7 cm margin to create the CTV. The positive lymph nodes in the pelvis (PLN) and para-aortic region (PALN) were defined on the fused FDG-PET/CT scan to create an MTV$_{nodal}$. An additional 0.7 cm margin was added to the CTV to create a PTV$_{PLN+PALN}$. The primary tumor in the cervix, MTV$_{cervix}$ was also defined on the fused images, including voxels with counts greater than 40% of the SUV$_{max}$. All subjects received high dose rate brachytherapy of 39 Gy in 6 fractions. The goal prescription doses were of 60 Gy, 50 Gy and 20 Gy in 30 fractions to the MTV$_{nodal}$, PTV$_{PLN+PALN}$, and MTV$_{cervix}$, respectively and were achieved in all 10 subjects. DVH analysis indicated that approximately 50% of the bowel received more than 25 Gy but also that less than 10% received below 50 Gy. DVHs of the kidney showed that approximately half of them received more than 16 Gy.[76,77]

Emerging Radiation Techniques

As previously outlined, approximately one-third of patients with locally advanced cervical cancer will have recurrent disease following standard therapy. In a substantial number of patients recurrence will include a pelvic component. Historically, patients with isolated local failure in the central pelvis have been previously considered for exenteration, a morbid procedure which can, however, offer cure. FDG-PET/CT can be of clinical use in these patients for ruling out other occult metastases before salvage therapy. A report by Chung and colleagues[78] showed that 40% of subjects with asymptomatic pelvic recurrence and no FDG-PET evidence of distant metastases were cured with exenteration.

In patients who are not candidates for curative surgery, outcomes are dismal with a 5-year overall survival of 3%.[79] Recently, stereotactic body radiation therapy (SBRT) has been evaluated as a salvage tool in patients with pelvic recurrence of gynecologic cancers who are not surgical candidates.[80,81] SBRT is an established technique for treatment of localized lung and liver tumors, with local control rates of 90% to 95%. It can deliver focal and conformal radiation doses with steep dose gradients toward normal tissue with subcentimeter accuracy.[82–87] Guckenberger and colleagues[80] reported their experience with SBRT in 19 subjects with unresectable, locally recurrent gynecologic cancers. They found a 3-year local control rate of 81%, which was, however, associated with 25% late GI toxicity. Additional studies have assessed the use of SBRT to treat isolated para-aortic recurrences of gynecologic cancers.[88]

FDG-PET/CT can be of clinical use in nonsurgical patients with recurrent cervical cancer by precisely delineating the volume of the relapsed tumor to allow dose escalation while sparing normal tissues. In addition, PET/CT can also identify occult metastases that may change the intent of therapy. In view of the high rate of local failure and its resultant morbidity, this emerging technique warrants further investigation in the subset of patients presenting with locally advanced disease.

FOLLOW-UP OF CERVICAL CANCER

Response to treatment is of prognostic value in patients with cervical cancer. Clinical assessment of response is challenging because after completion of radiotherapy most patients may still complain of pain, present with discharge, and urinary or gastrointestinal symptoms. Tumor volume assessed by physical examination does not necessarily indicate the presence of active disease. Serial FDG-PET studies performed during and up to 3 months after treatment of cervical cancer indicated that although most subjects achieved complete metabolic response by the end of treatment, abnormal FDG uptake post-therapy can predict tumor recurrence and death (**Fig. 4**).[89] Subjects with no FDG uptake 3 months after treatment had an actuarial 5-year recurrence-free survival of 83% compared with 0% in subjects with evidence of residual disease.[89] Furthermore, after treatment FDG uptake can vary across different regions of the cervical tumor volume. Intratumoral metabolic heterogeneity may be related to hypoxia and indicate a worse clinical outcome.[90]

There is no universally accepted follow-up approach in patients with cervical cancer. Although cytologic evaluation has been most commonly advocated along with clinical examination, retrospective studies by Zola and colleagues[91] and Bodurka-Bevers and colleagues[92] have shown

A

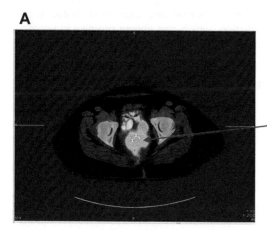

Cervix Tumor at Diagnosis with gold seed fudicial markers

B

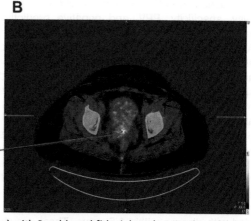

Negative 3-Month Post Therapy Cervix with gold seed fudicial markers

Fig. 4. (A) PET/CT showing FDG-avid cervical mass (*red arrow*) with 3 gold seed fiducial markers in place. (B) Post-treatment FDG-PET/CT study of the same patient as showing complete resolution of the previously noted FDG-PET avid cervical mass (*red arrow*) with residual gold seed fiducial markers.

that cytologic screening detected 0% and 3% of recurrent cervical cancer in asymptomatic subjects. In addition, in a retrospective review Morice and colleagues[93] showed that only 1 of 7 asymptomatic subjects were diagnosed by cytologic screening. Most studies have consistently shown that asymptomatic subjects with recurrent cervical cancer have a statistically significant higher overall survival.[91–93] Although this advantage could be caused by lead time bias, these results suggest that diagnostic techniques that can detect early, asymptomatic recurrence may be of clinical benefit.

Schwarz and colleagues[89] have assessed a prospective cohort of 92 subjects with cervical cancer stages IB1 to IVA who underwent pretreatment FDG-PET followed by chemoradiation. All subjects subsequently underwent a posttreatment FDG-PET study at a median 3-months interval. Based on the posttreatment FDG study results classified as complete metabolic response, partial response, or appearance of new abnormal tracer-avid foci, there were distinct differences in 3-year cause-specific survival rates of 96%, 43%, and 14%, respectively (P<.001). Furthermore, the hazard ratio for progression-free survival was 32.57 (95% confidence interval [CI], 10.22–103.82, P<.001) in subjects with tumor progression or recurrence and 6.30 (95%CI, 2.73–14.56; P<.001) for partial responders, compared with a hazard ratio of 3.54 (95%CI, 1.54–8.09; P = .003) for defining the pretreatment nodal status.

Multiple additional studies have demonstrated the value of FDG-PET in the follow-up of subjects with cervical cancer treated with definitive radiation, with and without chemotherapy.[79,94–98] A retrospective series by Ryu and colleagues,[95] including asymptomatic subjects, who performed surveillance FDG-PET studies showed a sensitivity, specificity, PPV, and negative predictive value of 90%, 76%, 35%, and 98%, respectively. Another series evaluating both symptomatic and asymptomatic subjects was published by Unger and colleagues[97] who reported a sensitivity and specificity of FDG-PET for detecting recurrence of 80% and 100% in asymptomatic and 100% and 86% in symptomatic subjects. Additionally, Singh and colleagues[99] evaluated 14 subjects with isolated para-aortic recurrences. Seven of the subjects with asymptomatic recurrence received chemoradiation and had an overall survival rate of 100%. The additional 7 symptomatic subjects did not receive chemoradiation and died with disease within 1.5 years. These results are consistent with a previous study of Grigsby and colleagues[100] who reported a 0% 2-year survival in 20, primarily symptomatic subjects with isolated PALN recurrence diagnosed by conventional imaging.

SUMMARY

Despite significant advances, cervical cancer continues to be a major worldwide public health concern. Although no randomized trials have directly compared FDG imaging to surgical staging, there is substantial evidence supporting its clinical utility in the management of patients with cervical cancer. The robust data has lead the National Comprehensive Cancer Network to recommend FDG imaging as part of the pretreatment assessment in cervical cancer with clinical stage IB2 or higher and to its further approval by the United States Center for Medicare and Medicaid Services.

Early asymptomatic local recurrences in the cervix, PLN, and PALN are readily detected on posttreatment FDG-PET/CT and have been associated with improved survival. FDG-PET/CT provides precise information on the MTV and these data have been instrumental in developing more advanced radiation treatment techniques, such as image-guided IMRT. This metabolic imaging modality will be instrumental in emerging treatment techniques, such as stereotactic body radiation, which has shown promise in unresectable local recurrent cervical cancer.

REFERENCES

1. Benedet JL, Bender H, Jones H III, et al. FIGO staging classifications and clinical practice guidelines in the management of gynecological cancers. Int J Gynecol Cancer 2000;70:221–9.
2. Jemal A, Siegel R, Ward E, et al. Cancer statistics, 2009. CA Cancer J Clin 2009;59:225–49.
3. Perez CA, Kavanagh BD. Cervical cancer. In: Halperin EC, Perez CA, Brady LW, editors. Perez and Brady's principle and practice of radiation oncology. 5th edition. Philadelphia: Lippincott Williams & Wilkins; 2008. p. 1533–600.
4. Eifel PJ, Winter K, Morris M, et al. Pelvic irradiation with concurrent chemotherapy versus pelvic and para-aortic irradiation for high-risk cervical cancer: an update of radiation therapy oncology group trial (RTOG) 90-01. J Clin Oncol 2004;22:872–80.
5. Keys HM, Bundy BN, Stehman FB, et al. Cisplatin, radiation, and adjuvant hysterectomy for bulky stage IB cervical carcinoma. N Engl J Med 1999; 340:1154–61.
6. Morris M, Eifel PJ, Lu J, et al. Pelvic radiation with concurrent chemotherapy compared with pelvic

and paraaortic radiation for high-risk cervical cancer. N Engl J Med 1999;340:1137–43.

7. Rose G, Bundy B, Watkins EB, et al. Concurrent cisplatin-based radiotherapy and chemotherapy for locally advanced cervical cancer. N Engl J Med 1999;340:1144–53.

8. Whitney CW, Sause W, Bundy BN, et al. A randomized comparison of fluorouracil plus cisplatin versus hydroxyurea as an adjunct to radiation therapy in stages IIB–IVA carcinoma of the cervix with negative para-aortic lymph nodes: a Gynecologic Oncology Group and Southwest Oncology Group Study. J Clin Oncol 1999;17: 1339–48.

9. Mitchell DG, Snyder B, Coakley F, et al. Early Invasive cervical cancer: tumor delineation by magnetic resonance imaging, computed tomography and clinical examination, verified by pathologic results, in ACRIN 6651/GOG 183 Intergroup Study. J Clin Oncol 2006;24:5687–94.

10. Grigsby PW, Dehdashti F, Siegel BA. FDG-PET evaluation of carcinoma of the cervix. Clin Positron Imaging. 1999;2:105–9.

11. Sironi S, Buda A, Picchio M, et al. Lymph node metastasis in patients with clinical early-stage cervical cancer: detection with integrated FDG PET/CT. Radiology 2006;238:272–9.

12. Averette HE, Ford JH, Dudan RC, et al. Staging of cervical cancer. Clin Obstet Gynecol 1975;18: 215–32.

13. van Nagel JR, Roddick JW, Lowin DM. The staging of cervical cancer: Inevitable discrepancies between clinical staging and pathologic findings. Am J Obstet Gynecol 1971;110:973–8.

14. Hricak H, Lacey C, Sandles LG, et al. Invasive cervical carcinoma: comparison of MR imaging and surgical findings. Radiology 1988;166:623–31.

15. Lagasse LD, Creasman WT, Shingleton HM, et al. Results and complications of operative staging in cervical cancer: experience of the Gynecologic Oncology Group. Gynecol Oncol 1980;9:90–8.

16. Bipat S, Glas AS, van der Velden J, et al. Computed tomography and magnetic resonance imaging in staging of uterine cervical carcinoma: a systematic review. Gynecol Oncol. 2003;91: 59–66.

17. Lanza A, Re A, D'Addato F, et al. Lymph nodal metastases and the clinical stage of cervix carcinoma. Eur J Gynaecol Oncol 1987;8:61–7.

18. Morice P, Sabourin JC, Pautie P, et al. Isolated para-aortic node involvement in stage Ib/II cervical carcinoma. Eur J Gynaecol Oncol 2000;21:123–5.

19. Deppe G, Lubicz S, Galloway BT, et al. Aortic node metastases with negative pelvic nodes in cervical cancer. Cancer 1984;53:173–5.

20. Trimble E. Cervical cancer state-of-the-clinical-science meeting on pretreatment evaluation and prognostic factors, September 27–28, 2007: proceedings and recommendations. Gynecol Oncol 2009;114:145–50.

21. Walsh JW, Goplerud DR. Prospective comparison between clinical and CT staging in primary cervical carcinoma. AJR Am J Roentgenol 1981;137: 997–1003.

22. Whitley NO, Brenner DE, Francis A, et al. Computed tomographic evaluation of carcinoma of the cervix. Radiology 1982;142:439–46.

23. Vick CW, Walsh JW, Wheelock JB, et al. CT of the normal and abnormal parametria in cervical cancer. AJR Am J Roentgenol 1984;143:597–603.

24. Hricak H, Phillips TL. Editorial on "The influence of tumor size and morphology on the outcome of patients with FIGO stage IB squamous cell carcinoma of the uterine cervix". Int J Radiat Oncol Biol Phys 1994;29:201–3.

25. Hricak H, Powell CB, Yu KK, et al. Invasive cervical carcinoma: role of MR imaging in pre-treatment work-up—cost minimization and diagnostic efficacy analysis. Radiology 1996;198:403–9.

26. Burghardt E, Hofmann HM, Ebner F, et al. Magnetic resonance imaging in cervical cancer: A basis for objective classification. Gynecol Oncol 1989;33: 61–7.

27. Hofmann HM, Ebner F, Haas J, et al. Magnetic resonance imaging in clinical cervical cancer: pre-therapeutic tumour volumetry. Baillieres Clin Obstet Gynaecol. 1988;2:789–802.

28. Greco A, Mason P, Leung AW, et al. Staging of carcinoma of the uterine cervix: MRI-surgical correlation. Clin Radiol 1989;40:401–5.

29. Mayr NA, Yuh WTC, Eng J, et al. Tumor size evaluated by pelvic examination compared with 3D MR quantitative analysis in the prediction of outcome for cervical cancer. Int J Radiat Oncol Biol Phys 1997;39:395–404.

30. Matsukuma K, Tsukamoto N, Matsuyama T, et al. Preoperative CT study of lymph nodes in cervical cancer: its correlation with histological findings. Gynecol Oncol 1989;33:168–71.

31. Kim SH, Choi BI, Lee HP, et al. Uterine cervical carcinoma: comparison of CT and MR findings. Radiology 1990;175:45–51.

32. Kim SH, Choi BI, Han JK, et al. Preoperative staging of uterine cervical carcinoma: comparison of CT and MR imaging in 99 patients. J Comput Assist Tomogr 1993;17:633–40.

33. Kim SH, Kim SC, Choi BI, et al. Uterine cervical carcinoma: evaluation of pelvic lymph node metastasis with MR imaging. Radiology 1994;190: 807–11.

34. Scheidler J, Hricak H, Yu KK, et al. Radiological evaluation of lymph node metastases in patients with cervical cancer: a meta-analysis. JAMA 1997;278:1096–101.

35. Hawighorst H, Schoenberg SO, Knapstein PG, et al. Staging of invasive cervical carcinoma and of pelvic lymph nodes by high resolution MR imaging with a phased-array coil in comparison with pathological findings. J Comput Assist Tomogr 1998;22:75–81.

36. Kaur H, Silverman PM, Iyer RB, et al. Diagnosis, staging, and surveillance of cervical carcinoma. AJR Am J Roentgenol 2003;180:1621–31.

37. Yang WT, Lam WM, Yu MY, et al. Comparison of dynamic helical CT and dynamic MR imaging in the evaluation of pelvic lymph nodes in cervical carcinoma. AJR Am J Roentgenol 2000;175:759–66.

38. Subak LL, Hricak H, Powell CB, et al. Cervical carcinoma: computed tomography and magnetic resonance imaging for preoperative staging. Obstet Gynecol 1995;86:43–50.

39. Williams AD, Cousins C, Soutter WP, et al. Detection of pelvic lymph node metastases in gynecologic malignancy: a comparison of CT, MR imaging, and positron emission tomography. Am J Roentgenol 2001;177:343–8.

40. Grigsby PW, Siegel BA, Dehdashti F. Lymph node staging by positron emission tomography in patients with carcinoma of the cervix. J Clin Oncol. 2001;19:3745–9.

41. Lewis P, Griffin S, Marsden P, et al. Whole-body 18F-fluorodeoxyglucose positron emission tomography in preoperative evaluation of lung cancer. Lancet 1994;344:1265–6.

42. Fleming ID, Cooper JS, Henson DE, et al. Staging of esophageal cancer with FDG-PET. AJR Am J Roentgenol 1997;168:417–24.

43. Rigo P, Paulus P, Kaschten BJ, et al. Oncological applications of PET. Eur J Nucl Med 1996;23:1641–74.

44. Block MI, Sundaresan SR, Patterson GA, et al. Improvement in staging of esophageal cancer with the addition of positron emission testing tomography. Ann Thorac Surg 1996;64:770–7.

45. Flanagan FL, Dehdashti F, Ogunbiyi OA, et al. Utility of FDG-PET for investigating unexplained plasma CEA elevation in patients with colorectal cancer. Ann Surg 1998;227:319–23.

46. Adler LP, Crowe JP, Al-Kaisi NK, et al. Evaluation of breast masses and axillary lymph nodes with [F18] 2-deoxy-2-fluoro-d-glucose PET. Radiology 1993;187:743–50.

47. Rose PG, Adler LP, Rodriguez M, et al. Positron emission tomography for evaluating para-aortic nodal metastasis in locally advanced cervical cancer before surgical staging: a surgicopathologic study. J Clin Oncol 1999;17:41–5.

48. Wong TZ, Jones EL, Coleman RE. Positron emission tomography with 2-deoxy-2-[(18)F]fluoro-D-glucose for evaluating local and distant disease in patients with cervical cancer. Mol Imaging Biol. 2004;6:55–62.

49. Showalter TN, Miller TM, Huettner P, et al. 18F-Fluorodeoxyglucose positron emission tomography and pathologic tumor size in early-stage invasive cervical cancer. Int J Gynecol Cancer 2009;19:1412–4.

50. Grigsby PW, Siegel BA, Dehdashti F, et al. Posttherapy [18F] fluorodeoxyglucose positron emission tomography in carcinoma of the cervix: response and outcome. J Clin Oncol 2004;22:2167–71.

51. Miller TR, Pinkus E, Dehdashti F, et al. Improved prognostic value of 18F-FDG PET using a simple visual analysis of tumor characteristics in patients with cervical cancer. J Nucl Med 2003;44:192–7.

52. Miller TR, Grigsby PW. Measurement of tumor volume by PET to evaluate prognosis in patients with advanced cervical cancer treated by radiation therapy. Int J Radiat Oncol Biol Phys 2002;53:353–9.

53. Singh AK, Grigsby PW, Dehdashti F, et al. FDG-PET lymph node staging and survival of patients with FIGO Stage IIIB cervical carcinoma. Int J Radiat Oncol Biol Phys 2003;56:489–93.

54. Stehman F, Bundy B, DiSaia P, et al. Carcinoma of the cervix treated with irradiation therapy. A multivariate analysis of prognostic variables in the Gynecologic Oncology Group. Cancer 1991;67:2776–85.

55. Kidd EA, Siegel BA, Dehdashti F, et al. Pelvic lymph node F-18 fluorodeoxyglucose uptake as a prognostic biomarker in newly diagnosed patients with locally advanced cervical cancer. Cancer 2007;110:1738–44.

56. Yen TC, See LC, Lai CH, et al. Standardized uptake value in para-aortic lymph nodes is a significant prognostic factor in patients with primary advanced squamous cervical cancer. Eur J Nucl Med Mol Imaging. 2008;35:493–501.

57. Borst GR, Belderbos JS, Boellaard R, et al. Standardised FDG uptake: a prognostic factor for inoperable non-small cell lung cancer. Eur J Cancer. 2005;41:1533–41.

58. Downey RJ, Akhurst T, Gonen M, et al. Preoperative F-18 fluorodeoxyglucose-positron emission tomography maximal standardized uptake value predicts survival after lung cancer resection. J Clin Oncol 2004;22:3255–60.

59. Eschmann SM, Friedel G, Paulsen F, et al. Is standardized (18)F-FDG uptake value an outcome predictor in patients with stage III non-small cell lung cancer? Eur J Nucl Med Mol Imaging 2006;33:263–9.

60. Pillot G, Siegel BA, Govindan R. Prognostic significance of fluorodeoxyglucose positron emission tomography in nonsmall cell lung cancer: a review. J Thorac Oncol 2006;1:152–9.

61. Sachs S, Bilfinger TV, Komaroff E, et al. Increased standardized uptake value in the primary lesion predicts nodal or distant metastases at presentation in lung cancer. Clin Lung Cancer 2005;6:310–3.

62. Belhocine T, Thille A, Fridman V, et al. Contribution of whole body 18FDG PET imaging in the management of cervical cancer. Gynecol Oncol 2002;87:90–7.

63. Reinhardt MJ, Ehritt-Braun C, Vogelgesang D, et al. Metastatic lymph nodes in patients with cervical cancer: detection with MR imaging and FDG PET. Radiology 2001;218:776–82.

64. Havrilesky LJ, Kulasingam SL, Matchar DB, et al. FDG-PET for management of cervical and ovarian cancer. Gynecol Oncol 2005;97:183–91.

65. Wright JD, Dehdashti F, Herzog TJ, et al. Preoperative lymph node staging of early-stage cervical carcinoma by [18F]-fluoro-2-deoxy-D-glucose-positron emission tomography. Cancer 2005;104:2484–91.

66. Tran BN, Grigsby PW, Dehdashti F, et al. Occult supraclavicular lymph node metastasis identified by FDG-PET in patients with carcinoma of the uterine cervix. Gynecol Oncol 2003;90:572–6.

67. Kidd EA, Siegel BA, Dehdashti F, et al. Pelvic lymph node F-18 fluorodeoxyglucose uptake as a prognostic biomarker in newly diagnosed patients with locally advanced cervical cancer. Cancer 2010;116:1469–75.

68. Reinstein LE, Wang XH, Burman CM, et al. A feasibility study of inverse treatment planning for cancer of the prostate. Int J Radiat Oncol Biol Phys 1998;40:207–14.

69. Verellen D, Linthout N, van den Berge D, et al. Initial experience with intensity-modulated conformal radiation therapy for the treatment of the head and neck region. Int J Radiat Oncol Biol Phys 1997;39:99–114.

70. Roeske JC, Lujan A, Rotmensch J, et al. Intensity-modulated whole pelvic radiation therapy in patients with gynecologic malignancies. Int J Radiat Oncol Biol Phys 2000;48:1613–21.

71. Mundt AJ, Lujan AE, Rotmensch J, et al. Intensity-modulated whole pelvic radiotherapy in women with gynecologic malignancies. Int J Radiat Oncol Biol Phys 2002;52:1330–7.

72. Mundt AJ, Mell LK, Roeske JC. Preliminary analysis of chronic gastrointestinal toxicity in gynecology patients treated with intensity-modulated whole pelvic radiation therapy. Int J Radiat Oncol Biol Phys 2003;56:1354–60.

73. Portelance L, Chao KS, Grigsby PW, et al. Intensity-modulated radiation therapy (IMRT) reduces small bowel, rectum, and bladder doses in patients with cervical cancer receiving pelvic and para-aortic irradiation. Int J Radiat Oncol Biol Phys 2001;51:261–6.

74. Salama JK, Mundt AJ, Roeske J, et al. Preliminary outcome and toxicity report of extended-field, intensity-modulated radiation therapy for gynecologic malignancies. Int J Radiat Oncol Biol Phys 2006;65:1170–6.

75. Macdonald DM, Lin LL, Biehl K, et al. Combined intensity-modulation radiation therapy and brachytherapy in the treatment of cervical cancer. Int J Radiat Oncol Biol Phys 2008;71:618–24.

76. Esthappan J, Chaudhuri S, Santanam L, et al. Prospective clinical trial of positron emission tomography/computed tomography radiation therapy for cervical carcinoma with positive para-aortic lymph nodes. Int J Radiat Oncol Biol Phys 2008;72:1134–9.

77. Esthappan J, Mutic S, Malyapa RS, et al. Treatment planning guidelines regarding the use of CT/PET-guided IMRT for cervical carcinoma with positive paraaortic lymph nodes. Int J Radiat Oncol Biol Phys 2004;58:1289–97.

78. Chung HH, Kim SK, Kim TH, et al. Clinical impact of FDG-PET imaging in post-therapy surveillance of uterine cervical cancer: from diagnosis to prognosis. Gynecol Oncol 2006;103:165–70.

79. Hong JH, Tsai CS, Lai CH, et al. Recurrent squamous cell carcinoma of cervix after definitive radiotherapy. Int J Radiat Oncol Biol Phys 2004;60:249–57.

80. Guckenberger M, Bachmann J, Wulf J, et al. Stereotactic body radiation therapy for local boost therapy in unfavourable locally recurrent gynaecological cancer. Radiother Oncol 2010;94:53–9.

81. Kunos C, Chen W, DeBernardo R, et al. Stereotactic body radiosurgery for pelvic relapse of gynecologic malignancies. Tech Canc Res Treat 2009;8:393–400.

82. Schefter TE, Cardenes HR, Kavanagh. Stereotactic body radiation therapy for liver tumors. In: Kavanagh B, Timmerman RD, editors. Stereotactic body radiation therapy. 1st edition. Baltimore (MD): Lippincott, Williams, and Wilkins; 2005. p. 115–24.

83. Song DY, Blomgren H. Stereotactic body radiation therapy for lung tumors. In: Kavanagh B, Timmerman RD, editors. Stereotactic body radiation therapy. 1st edition. Baltimore: Lippincott, Williams, and Wilkins; 2005. p. 99–107.

84. Wulf J, Oppitz U, Thiele W, et al. Stereotactic radiotherapy for primary lung cancer and pulmonary metastases: a noninvasive treatment approach in medically inoperable patients. Int J Radiat Oncol Biol Phys 2004;60:186–96.

85. Lax I, Naslund I, Näslund I, et al. Stereotactic radiotherapy of malignancies in the abdomen: methodological aspects. Acta Oncol 1994;33:677–83.

86. Potters L, Rose C, Timmerman R, et al. American Society for Therapeutic Radiology and Oncology; American College of Radiology practice guideline

for the performance of stereotactic body radiation therapy. Int J Radiat Oncol Biol Phys 2004;60: 1026–32.

87. Timmerman R, McGarry R, Likes L, et al. Extracranial stereotactic radioablation: results of a phase I study in medically inoperable stage I non-small cell lung cancer. Chest 2003;124:1946–55.

88. Choi CW, Cho CK, Yoo SY, et al. Image-guided stereotactic body radiation therapy in patients with isolated para-aortic lymph node metastases from uterine cervical and corpus cancer. Int J Radiat Oncol Biol Phys 2009;74:147–53.

89. Schwarz JK, Siegel BA, Dehdashti F, et al. The association of posttherapy positron emission tomography with tumor response and survival in cervical carcinoma. JAMA 2007;298:2289–95.

90. Grigsby PW. The prognostic value of PET and PET/CT in cervical cancer. Cancer Imaging. 2008;8: 146–55.

91. Zola P, Fuso L, Mazzola S, et al. Follow-up strategies in gynecological oncology: searching appropriateness. Int J Gynecol Cancer 2007;17: 1186–93.

92. Bodurka-Bevers D, Morris M, Eifel P, et al. Posttherapy surveillance of women with cervical cancer: an outcomes analysis. Gynecol Oncol 2000;78: 187–93.

93. Morice P, Deyrolle C, Rey A, et al. Value of routine follow-up procedures for patients with stage I/II cervical cancer treated with combined surgery-radiation therapy. Ann Oncol 2004;15:218–23.

94. Brooks RA, Rader JS, Dehdashti F, et al. Surveillance FDG-PET detection of asymptomatic recurrences in patients with cervical cancer. Gynecol Oncol 2009;112:104–9.

95. Ryu SY, Kim MH, Choi SC, et al. Detection of early recurrence with 18F-FDG PET in patients with cervical cancer. J Nucl Med 2003;44:347–52.

96. Havrilesky LJ, Wong TZ, Secord AA, et al. The role of PET scanning in the detection of recurrent cervical cancer. Gynecol Oncol 2003;90: 186–90.

97. Unger JB, Ivy JJ, Connor P, et al. Detection of recurrent cervical cancer by whole-body FDG PET scan in asymptomatic and symptomatic women. Gynecol Oncol 2004;94:212–6.

98. Kitajima K, Murakami K, Yamasaki E, et al. Performance of FDG-PET/CT for diagnosis of recurrent uterine cervical cancer. Eur Radiol 2008;18: 2040–7.

99. Singh AK, Grigsby PW, Rader JS, et al. Cervix carcinoma, concurrent chemotherapy, and salvage of isolated paraaortic lymph node recurrence. Int J Radiat Oncol Biol Phys 2005;61:450–5.

100. Grigsby PW, Vest M, Perez C. Recurrent carcinoma of the cervix exclusively in the para-aortic nodes following radiation therapy. Int J Radiat Oncol Biol Phys 1994;28:451–5.

The Roles of Fluorodeoxyglucose-PET/Computed Tomography in Ovarian Cancer: Diagnosis, Assessing Response, and Detecting Recurrence

Richard L. Wahl, MD[a,c,*], Mehrbod Som Javadi, MD[a],
Hedieh Eslamy, MD[a], Aditi Shruti, MD[a],
Robert Bristow, MD[b,c]

KEYWORDS

• Fluorodeoxyglucose • PET • Computed tomography
• Ovarian cancer

Ovarian cancer has the highest mortality of all gynecologic cancers, despite representing only 3% of all cancers in women. About 21,550 new cases of ovarian cancer and an estimated 14,600 deaths caused by this cancer occurred in the United States in 2009.[1] Patients who have ovarian cancer often present with advanced disease resulting in a high mortality.

At present, about 90% of ovarian cancers are judged as sporadic. About 10% of ovarian cancers are autosomal inherited forms: site-specific ovarian cancer; and hereditary breast and/or ovarian cancer, of which about 90% are caused by BRCA-1 and BRCA-2 gene mutations and about 10% caused by Lynch syndrome, formerly known as hereditary nonpolyposis colorectal cancer syndrome mutations in mismatch repair genes MLH1, MSH2, MSH6, PMS2, which are susceptibility genes for Lynch syndrome.[2] Relative risks of cancer of 20- to 45-fold in the general population have been described for carriers of these mutations. Not all patients with the mutations develop cancer, but up to 50% often do, and many of them occur before the menopause. Risk-reducing salpingo-oophorectomy has been applied in an effort to reduce the probability of a new cancer developing.[3] This approach is increasingly favored, because the use of screening ultrasound (US) has not proven sufficiently sensitive to exclude ovarian cancers from presenting at an advanced stage.[2] Part of the challenge in screening is that a significant portion of the cancers develop on the serosa and thus can disseminate intraperitoneally early while the tumors are small. A small percentage of ovarian cancers develop from the peritoneum, so prophylactic oophorectomy is not 100% successful in preventing ovarian cancer occurrence.

[a] Division of Nuclear Medicine, Johns Hopkins University School of Medicine, Baltimore, MD, USA
[b] Division of Gynecological Oncology, Johns Hopkins University School of Medicine, Baltimore, MD, USA
[c] Division of Oncology, Johns Hopkins University School of Medicine, Baltimore, MD, USA
* Corresponding author. Division of Nuclear Medicine, Johns Hopkins University School of Medicine, Baltimore, MD.
E-mail address: rwahl@jhmi.edu

PET Clin 5 (2010) 447–461
doi:10.1016/j.cpet.2010.07.008
1556-8598/10/$ — see front matter © 2010 Published by Elsevier Inc.

Histologically, ovarian cancers are differentiated by the cell of origin: epithelial (90%), and stromal, germ cell, or mixed for the remainder.

Ovarian cancer results in regional and distant spread through 4 main pathways[1]: penetration of the ovarian capsule and direct invasion of contiguous organs or the pelvic peritoneum,[2] spread via the lymphatic system to the pelvic and paraaortic lymph nodes,[3] penetration of ovarian capsule and subsequent peritoneal spread, and[4] hematogenous spread.[3,4]

There are several possible diagnostic tasks for [18F]fluorodeoxyglucose (FDG)-PET imaging in ovarian cancer, including noninvasive characterization of an ovarian mass as malignant or benign imaging; early diagnosis and defining the extent of localized ovarian cancer; staging and initial treatment planning (which often includes debulking surgery) after the diagnosis, predicting whether response will occur and determining whether the disease is responding to treatment; determining whether there is residual tumor (restaging) or recurrence after the treatment, critical diagnostic points because the treatments for ovarian cancer can be aggressive and difficult for patients to tolerate. FDG-PET has been evaluated to some extent in each of these settings, but the role of PET in detecting recurrent disease and in monitoring response to tumors are the major areas of focus of this article.

CLINICAL BACKGROUND
Primary Disease Detection

A robust method to screen for ovarian cancer has the potential to reduce mortality from this disease, much as has occurred with cervical cancer and the use of cytologic staining. To date, a single modality screening method for ovarian cancer using either blood measurements of the tumor marker CA-125 or transvaginal ultrasonography (TVS) has not provided the accuracy necessary for reliable, cost-effective, early detection of this cancer. Multimodality screening using serum CA-125 and pelvic US or TVS seems to improve the median survival in the screened group.[5–8] Currently there are at least 2 large ongoing trials for multimodal screening (CA-125 and TVS) in ovarian cancer. The final assessment of the accuracy of such approaches will have to await the analysis of the complete cohort and longer follow-up to assess the effect on mortality.[9,10] Such studies can identify patients with ovarian masses that then need further workup. However, high false-positive rates and adverse outcomes from false-positive studies diminish the usefulness of screening approaches in women at high risk.

Most ovarian masses in premenopausal women are benign and functionally related to the menstrual cycle. When incidentally detected, these masses are typically followed for regression by physical examination or US. Premenopausal women can develop ovarian cancer, and a mass that does not resolve or regress in such a patient is of considerable concern for cancer and requires further workup because of a greater probability of malignancy. By contrast, ovarian masses in postmenopausal women are commonly malignant and far more concerning for cancer than masses in the premenopausal woman.

Morphologic imaging may be used to characterize adnexal masses as benign or malignant and delineate regional or distant spread before surgery. In a recent meta-analysis, Liu and colleagues[11] compared the performance of US, computed tomography (CT) and magnetic resonance (MR) imaging in differentiation of malignant from benign ovarian tumors. Sensitivity estimates of all imaging modalities were comparable: 89% (95% confidence interval [CI] 88%–90%) for US, 85% (95% CI 83%–86%) for CT, and 89% (95% CI 88%–92%) for MR ($P = .09$), as well as specificity estimates: 95% CI 83%–85% for US, 95% CI 76%–92% for CT, and 95% CI 84%–88% for MR ($P = .12$). The investigators concluded that morphologic assessment using US is still the most important and common modality in the detection of ovarian cancer. However, because none of these imaging methods achieve total accuracy, persistent ovarian masses in postmenopausal women are commonly surgically excised to avoid delayed diagnosis of ovarian carcinoma

Staging

Traditionally, ovarian cancer has been staged surgically. The tumor-node-metastasis (TNM) and International Federation of Gynecology and Obstetrics (FIGO) staging systems classify ovarian cancers as: stage I, tumor limited to ovaries (1 or both); stage II, tumor involving 1 or both ovaries with pelvic extension; stage III, tumor involving 1 or both ovaries with microscopic/macroscopic peritoneal metastases beyond the pelvis and/or regional lymph node metastases; stage IV, distant metastases (excluding peritoneal metastases).[12]

The FIGO criteria do not specify the mechanism of detection of stage IV disease. Essential elements of surgical staging of ovarian cancer include peritoneal cytology; intact tumor removal; complete abdominal exploration; removal of the remaining ovary, uterus, and fallopian tubes; infracolic omentectomy; pelvic and paraaortic lymph node sampling; and multiple biopsies, including blind biopsies from areas at risk for spread (ie, diaphragm, paracolic gutters, and pelvis). Prognosis is influenced by the diameter of the residual disease after primary cytoreductive surgery, with optimal and suboptimal debulking being defined as the largest diameter of a residual nodule as 1 cm or less or more than 1 cm, respectively. It is desirable to surgically reduce the tumor volume to the greatest extent possible in such procedures.[4]

Approximately 20% to 30% of patients with early-stage disease (stage IA–IIA) and 50% to 75% of those with advanced disease (stage IIB–IV) who achieve a complete response following first-line chemotherapy ultimately develop recurrent disease, which more frequently involves the pelvis and abdomen.[13]

In a recent study, preoperative CT and MR imaging were found to be reasonably accurate in the detection of inoperable tumor and in the prediction of suboptimal debulking for a sensitivity, specificity, positive predictive value (PPV), and negative predictive value (NPV) of 76%, 92%, 94%, and 96% respectively. The two modalities were equally effective ($P = 1.0$) in the detection of inoperable tumor. This study suggests that imaging may help triage inoperable patients to a more appropriate neoadjuvant chemotherapy group.[14] The sensitivity of 76% indicates that there are still major opportunities to improve imaging accuracy, especially for low tumor volume disease.

The standard of care for patients with ovarian carcinoma is primary cytoreductive surgery and, in patients with advanced disease who are not candidates for surgery, neoadjuvant chemotherapy is administered, typically paclitaxel and carboplatin (except in some stage IA and IB patients). Intraperitoneal (IP) therapies can be particularly effective, if tolerated.[15] A prospective trial in 415 patients showed that, for the patients who could tolerate the toxic IP therapy approach, the median duration of progression-free survival (PFS) and overall survival (OS) were significantly prolonged compared with patients who received intravenous chemotherapy (PFS of 23.8 vs 18.3 months, $P<.03$ and DFS 65.6 vs 49.7 months, $P<.05$ respectively).[16] Localized borderline histology tumors are sometimes not treated with chemotherapy.

Suspected Recurrence

Ovarian cancer primarily recurs in the peritoneal cavity and retroperitoneal lymph nodes. Patients are monitored for recurrence with periodic physical examinations, serum CA-125 level measurements, and US examinations. Additional imaging (CT, MR imaging, and FDG-PET or PET/CT) is commonly performed when there are signs or symptoms suggestive of recurrence.[4,13,17] However, both morphologic (CT and MR imaging) and metabolic FDG-PET imaging are limited in their ability to detect small-volume (<5–10 mm) disease. Rising CA-125 levels may precede the clinical detection of recurrence in 56% to 94% of cases, with a median lead time of 3 to 5 months.[13] Recent data suggest FDG-PET to be more sensitive than CA-125 levels, in some instances.

In the 1970s and 1980s, second-look laparotomy (SLL), defined as a comprehensive surgical exploration in an asymptomatic patient who has completed primary cytoreductive surgery and adjuvant chemotherapy, was widely used. SLL does not seem to have a role in the management of early-stage ovarian cancer and its role in patients with advanced-stage disease is controversial.[4]

Treatment options for recurrent ovarian cancer include salvage chemotherapy, experimental protocols, hormonal therapy, secondary cytoreductive surgery, and palliative and hospice care. The choice of the chemotherapeutic regimen depends on whether the disease is platinum sensitive or platinum resistant. Patients with disease progression while receiving platinum-based therapy, patients who fail to achieve a complete clinical response, and those who relapse within 6 months of the end of chemotherapy are classified as platinum resistant.[4,17] Initiation of treatment in patients with biochemical relapse (CA-125>35 U/mL or doubling of the post-treatment nadir level) and negative radiographic studies is a controversial topic, but is performed in some settings.[4,17]

ROLES OF FDG IMAGING IN OVARIAN CANCER

Ovarian cancers have been shown to be FDG avid in animal models, to express high levels of the glucose transporter Glut 1, and to have higher FDG uptake in areas of viable cancer than in normal tissues (including normal lymph nodes) in human xenograft studies. Pilot studies showing the feasibility of PET imaging of ovarian cancer were reported as early as 1991.[18,19]

Nearly all PET imaging of ovarian cancer is currently performed with FDG as the radiotracer. As with other FDG-avid cancers, patients should be imaged in the fasting state to minimize insulin levels and the targeting of FDG to normal insulin-responsive tissues such as skeletal muscle. The approach to imaging may vary slightly, depending on the individual PET center. In our institution, patient preparation for ovarian cancer imaging is similar to that for oncologic imaging in general, with fasting for at least 4 hours (and ideally overnight), with no specific urinary tract preparation. We normally use dilute positive oral contrast in our patients to achieve definitive positive bowel visualization. It is rare to use bladder irrigation or catheterization, but critically important for patients to be well hydrated and to void immediately before imaging. Another approach to dealing with urinary tract activity can be use of an additional delayed image after voiding if there is any confusion regarding the radiotracer activity levels in the urinary tract. Iterative reconstruction approaches are now used routinely. The proper uptake time from tracer injection until imaging has to be long enough for the FDG to accumulate avidly into the tumors, although the radiotracer can decay substantially. Most FDG imaging in ovarian cancer is started about 60 minutes after tracer injection, but longer delays of 90 minutes to 2 hours commonly result in superior target/background uptake ratios but lower total counts in the images. Dual time point imaging has been applied to a limited extent.[20] At our center, delayed images are obtained if there is uncertainty in the differential diagnosis of FDG-avid sites between excreted or physiologic tracer activity versus active tumor. FDG-PET and/or PET/CT in ovarian carcinoma has been considered and/or investigated to varying extents in settings that are discussed later.

FDG IMAGING IN SCREENING FOR PRIMARY OVARIAN CANCER

There have been no systematic studies of FDG-PET used specifically for detection of ovarian carcinoma in a screening setting. Radiation exposure with PET/CT is not minimal and exposure of large numbers of patients to ionizing radiation in a screening program may result in a high population radiation burden. FDG-PET is an expensive procedure and therefore screening would have to provide a high yield of cancer detection to be cost-effective. General cancer screening of patient populations without a markedly increased risk of cancer has detected only few ovarian cancers.[21] Moreover, large numbers of patients with known or suspected cancers are being imaged with FDG-PET for other reasons. Although a wide range of cancers have been detected in these series, with a prevalence of 1% to 2%, ovarian cancer has not been detected with any substantive frequency.[22] Given the radiation exposure from screening studies and the limited anecdotal data available, at present there is not an established role for PET screening in ovarian cancer.

FDG-PET/CT might serve as a useful adjunct to TVS in a high-risk population, perhaps to help characterize masses. Such high-risk groups are being increasingly defined, such as BRCA-1 and BRCA-2 mutant populations.

Increased ovarian radiotracer uptake in an asymptomatic woman being imaged for reasons other than ovarian carcinoma by FDG-PET/CT should be considered carefully.

Lerman and colleagues[23] reported increased ovarian FDG uptake in 21 of 119 premenopausal patients without known gynecologic malignancy. The investigators concluded that increased ovarian FDG uptake is associated with malignancy in postmenopausal patients but may be either functional or malignant in premenopausal patients. Although typically, in premenopausal women, ovarian FDG uptake is functional, such a finding requires additional clinical and imaging follow-up to confirm that the findings have resolved or are stable. Kim and colleagues[24] correlated the presence of incidental FDG accumulation in the ovary with the menstrual history, concurrent morphologic imaging (MR imaging, CT, and US), and surgical or imaging (PET or CT) follow-up in 19 patients who did not have a primary or metastatic ovarian malignancy. They concluded that the typical spherical or discoid FDG accumulation in the ovary during the luteal or ovulatory phase represents normal physiologic uptake in ovarian follicles or corpus lutei. A recent report from China had similar findings.[25] Thus, if incidental ovarian uptake is identified in a younger woman, it is more likely benign than malignant, but must be followed closely because cancer can also occur in premenopausal women. In postmenopausal women, such uptake is far more concerning for cancer. Appropriate follow-up can include pelvic US about 6 weeks later, or a repeat PET/CT study. Physical examination is insensitive for small lesions. Although it is possible to envision a role of FDG-PET in screening women at high risk of ovarian cancer, such as those with BRCA mutations, it is unlikely that such a program will become a first-line approach.

FDG IMAGING IN DIAGNOSIS OF PRIMARY OVARIAN CARCINOMA

Diagnosis differs from screening in that the task is differentiation of benign from malignant lesions in patients presenting with asymptomatic adnexal masses diagnosed either by physical examination, incidentally as a result of other imaging tests, or by screening programs. The original literature was generated using FDG-PET only, whereas essentially all recent studies have used PET/CT imaging.

Locations for the ovaries in the pelvis are complex and variable, and recent results with PET/CT have generally been more accurate than those with PET only.

The sensitivity for detection of ovarian cancer using PET is likely dependent on the lesion histology as well as the lesion size. Small lesions, less than 1 cm in size, are likely to be more difficult to detect than larger lesions because of the resolution limitations of current PET systems. Detection of microscopic disease is beyond the resolution of PET/CT systems. By contrast, the detection of macroscopic tumors before a treatment-induced reduction in glucose metabolism is more realistic and feasible.

US has been the modality of choice in the evaluation of patients with suspected adnexal masses, with MR imaging used in uncertain or problematic cases.[26] Hubner and colleagues[27] correlated the results of FDG-PET and CT imaging of ovarian masses with pathology. The calculated sensitivity, specificity, accuracy, PPV, and NPV were fair, 83%, 80%, 82%, 86%, and 76% for PET and 82%, 53%, 72%, 77%, and 62% for CT. Rieber and colleagues[28] prospectively compared the diagnostic performance of TVS, PET, and MR imaging in 103 patients with suspicious adnexal findings on US, in whom subsequent histology revealed 12 malignant and 91 benign ovarian tumors. The sensitivity, specificity, and accuracy were 58%, 78%, and 76% for PET; 83%, 84%, and 83% for MR imaging; 92%, 59%, and 63% for US; and 92%, 84%, and 85% for all 3 modalities in consensus. Kawahara and colleagues[29] prospectively compared MR imaging with FDG-PET in 38 patients suspected of having ovarian cancer based on findings from physical examination and US. Histology revealed 23 malignant and 15 benign lesions. The sensitivity, specificity, and accuracy were 78%, 87%, and 82% for PET, 91%, 87%, and 92% for MR imaging, and 91%, 87%, and 92% for the 2 modalities in consensus.

Combined PET/CT showed a higher sensitivity and specificity of 100% and 92.5% respectively ($P<.00005$) in the diagnosis of a malignant tumor in patients with a pelvic mass of unknown origin and increased risk of malignancy based on a substantially increased serum CA-125, US examinations, and the menopausal state.[30] The investigators suggested that PET/CT was the imaging modality of choice when US shows a pelvic tumor and additional information before surgery is needed. Borderline and benign tumors were both placed in the benign group in this study, which may not be suitable for routine management. Nam and colleagues[31] recently reported

on the use of PET/CT in 133 women suspected to have ovarian cancer, enrolled in a prospective study of PET/CT, MR imaging, and US, with surgery as a gold standard. Histopathology showed benign tumors in 25 patients, borderline lesions in 13 patients, and malignant tumors in 95 patients. In distinguishing malignant/borderline tumors from benign ovarian masses, the accuracy of PET/CT (92%) was higher than that of pelvic US (83%) and abdominopelvic CT or pelvic MR imaging (74%; $P = .013$). PET had a sensitivity of about 98% for cancer detection. The prevalence of ovarian cancer in this population is high, making the NPV of PET low.[31] Results from larger studies using PET/CT seem superior to those of PET as a stand-alone procedure. PET/CT seems superior to US and MR imaging for characterizing ovarian masses, although it is probable that US played a role in the patients referred to PET/CT imaging.[32] Even with a sensitivity of 95%, PET may be inadequate to preclude surgery in women with ovarian masses that persist. PET/CT could lead to observation or laparoscopy versus laparotomy in some subpopulations of women, although finite false-positive and false-negative rate means will maintain residual uncertainty in ovarian mass characterization, based on a single PET/CT study.

Some possible causes of false-positive and false-negative findings on FDG-PET in patients with adnexal masses are summarized in **Box 1**.

FDG IMAGING IN STAGING OF OVARIAN CANCER

Ovarian cancer has typical routes of distribution for metastases. The FIGO criteria do not specify the mechanism of detection of stage IV disease. Thus, a sensitive method such as FDG-PET likely detects more stage IV disease than a chest radiograph or physical examination, potentially resulting in upward stage migration in patients using PET. Most data indicate FDG-PET/CT to be the single most accurate method of staging ovarian cancer at the time of initial presentation. Results vary by study and by whether a lesion- or patient-based analysis has been conducted. Lesion-based analyses typically have lower sensitivities than patient-based studies. Yoshida and colleagues[33] prospectively evaluated the performance of FDG-PET/CT versus CT alone for the preoperative staging of 15 patients with suspected ovarian cancer by physical examination, sonography, and serum CA-125 levels. All patients underwent surgical staging within 2 weeks of the imaging examinations. The lesion-based sensitivity, specificity, accuracy, PPV, and NPV were 46%, 90%, 83%, 47%, and 90%

respectively for CT, and 68%, 92%, 88%, 65%, and 93% respectively for PET/CT. The patient-based diagnostic accuracy was 53% for CT and 78% for FDG-PET/CT. Peritoneal carcinomatosis, which can often be found in patients with ovarian cancer, can present as either focal or uniform FDG uptake, corresponding with nodular and diffuse peritoneal disease respectively on FDG scans, and deserves special consideration.[34]

In the large prospective study mentioned earlier, imaging PET/CT staging was concordant with surgical staging in 78% of patients. PET/CT further revealed 16% previously unknown extra-abdominal lymph node metastases in 95 patients. PET/CT was generally superior to MR imaging and CT (although these tests were not performed in each case) in detecting regional nodal metastases. In addition, PET/CT detected new, unexpected coexisting malignant tumors in 5 (3.8%) cases.[31] Kitajima and colleagues[35] evaluated the accuracy of integrated FDG-PET/CT with intravenous contrast (PET/ceCT) for preoperative staging of ovarian cancer, compared with enhanced CT, using surgical and histopathologic findings as the reference standard. Forty patients underwent FDG-PET/ceCT before primary debulking surgery.

The PET/CT and CT components were interpreted separately by 2 experienced radiologists by consensus. The results of the 2 modalities were concordant with the final pathologic staging in 55% and 75% of cases, respectively. The overall lesion-based (n = 680) sensitivity improved from 37.6% to 69.4%, the specificity from 97.1% to 97.5%, and the accuracy from 89.7% to 94.0% between CT and PET/CT. PET/ceCT was superior to enhanced CT in this primary staging setting. Again, both the PET and CT component failed to detect what were probably small lesions found at pathology.[35]

Two-hundred and one patients with a Risk of Malignancy Index greater than 150 based on serum CA-125, US examinations, and menopausal state underwent PET/CT within 2 weeks before standard surgery/debulking of a pelvic tumor, with data from 66 of the patients with ovarian cancer available for analysis. Fifty-one percent were diagnosed with PET/CT stage III and 41% with PET/CT stage IV disease. Survival was significantly longer for patients with PET/CT stage III than for patients with PET/CT stage IV ($P = .03$). Using univariate analysis, PET/CT stage III ($P = .03$), complete debulking (no macroscopic residual tumor) ($P = .002$), and Gynecologic Oncology Group performance status less than or equal to 2 ($P = .04$) were statistically significant prognostic variables. Using multivariate Cox regression analysis, complete debulking was the only statistically significant independent prognostic variable ($P = .02$). Thus, although FDG-PET/CT is of prognostic value after primary staging, it is not independent of the quality of debulking. PET may also lead to upstaging and stage migration by detecting smaller additional foci of tumor, although low-volume disease can fail to be detected on PET/CT.[36]

FDG IMAGING FOR RESTAGING OF OVARIAN CANCER

Despite adequate standard of treatment using cytoreductive surgery followed by platinum-based chemotherapy and complete response, recurrence is a major problem for ovarian cancer. It has been estimated that 60% of patients diagnosed in an advanced stage will develop abdominal relapse. Restaging is similar to initial staging. FDG-PET/CT has been used for evaluating patients with clinically suspected recurrence and/or for precise localization of extent of disease after treatment.

Many investigators have retrospectively or prospectively evaluated the diagnostic value of PET or PET/CT in patients with clinically suspected ovarian cancer recurrence based on symptoms, physical examination, serum tumor markers, or morphologic imaging, as well as in patients who are clinically disease free (ie, restaging vs surveillance). Because these 2 groups have potentially different pretest probabilities of a positive PET finding, they should be considered separately.

Restaging is typically performed either in patients with suspected tumor recurrence or in patients with documented tumor recurrence on anatomic imaging to accurately localize extent of disease for treatment planning. The effect of metabolic imaging restaging on patient management has been studied (Table 1).[37–43] Some of the early studies have a small sample size and therefore lack statistical power, and also use different standards of reference and different imaging methodologies (PET vs PET/CT vs PET/CT with intravenous contrast).

Bristow and colleagues[44] prospectively evaluated the usefulness of PET/CT in patient selection for secondary cytoreductive surgery. Their standard of reference was recurrent ovarian tumor measuring 1 cm or more at the time of surgery, a size associated with an optimal debulking procedure. This size cutoff for macroscopic disease is different from other studies that also considered microscopic disease and macroscopic disease of less than 1 cm in the calculation of sensitivity and specificity of PET. In this study, PET/CT had an estimated sensitivity of 81.8% and specificity of 83.3% in detecting recurrent disease of 1 cm or more. Bristow and colleagues[45] also retrospectively evaluated 14 patients with rising serum CA-125 levels, and negative or

equivocal conventional CT imaging 6 months or more after primary therapy. Eleven patients (78.6%) had recurrent ovarian cancer limited to retroperitoneal lymph nodes targeted by PET/CT and underwent surgical reassessment of targeted nodal basins. Of 143 nodes retrieved, 59 contained recurrent ovarian cancer (median nodal diameter 2.5 cm, range 0.8–5.2 cm). For all target nodal basins, the sensitivity, specificity, PPV, NPV, and accuracy for recurrent ovarian cancer in dissected lymph nodes were 40.7% (24/59), 94.0% (79/84), 82.8% (24/29), 69.3% (79/114), and 72.0% (103/143) ($P<.001$). PET/CT failed to identify microscopic disease in 59.3% of pathologically positive nodes. The investigators concluded that PET/CT shows a high PPV in identifying recurrent ovarian cancer in retroperitoneal lymph nodes when conventional CT findings are negative or equivocal. The high incidence of occult disease within the target nodal basins suggests that regional lymphadenectomy may be necessary for complete secondary cytoreduction of recurrent disease. These findings in lymph nodes are similar to those described in breast cancer, for which false-negative results in small tumor foci were not uncommon. In a small study from the same institution, Pannu and colleagues[46] showed a low sensitivity of PET/CT for lesions less than 1 cm in diameter (13%), again illustrating the limitations of PET/CT in low-volume disease. Sironi and colleagues[47] prospectively evaluated the accuracy of PET/CT for depicting persistent ovarian carcinoma after first-line treatment in 31 patients, with use of histologic findings as the reference standard. The overall lesion-based sensitivity, specificity, accuracy, PPV, and NPV

Table 1
Performance of FDG imaging for restaging of ovarian cancer

Author	Modality	N	Sensitivity (%)	Specificity (%)
Yen et al[37]	PET	24	91	92
Zimny et al[38]	PET	58	94	75
Nakamoto et al[39]	PET	12	80	50
Torizuka et al[40]	PET	25	80	100
Takekuma et al[41]	PET	29	84.6	100
Nanni et al[42]	PET/CT	41	88.2	71.4 (accuracy 85.4%)
Chung et al[43]	PET/CT	77	93.3	96.9
Bristow et al[44]	PET/CT	22	81.8 (in detecting recurrent disease ≥1 cm)	83.3
Sironi et al[47]	PET/CT	31	78	75
Thrall et al[57]	PET/CT	24	94	100
Sebastian et al[48]	PET/CT	53		Accuracy 94%
Risum et al[36]	PET/CT	60	97%	90

of PET/CT were 78%, 75%, 77%, 89%, and 57% respectively. All lesions missed on PET/CT were 0.5 cm or less in maximum diameter, again consistent with the limited ability of PET to detect microscopic disease.

PET/CT was recently compared with CT in detecting ovarian carcinoma recurrence in 51 consecutive patients who underwent 53 restaging PET/CT scans.[48] The accuracy of PET/CT exceeded that of CT for body (92% [49/53] versus 83% [44/53]), chest (96% [51/53] versus 89% [47/53]), and abdomen (91% [48/53] versus 79% [42/53]). PET was more accurate than CT in the abdomen by receiver operating characteristic analysis (P<.01). Interobserver agreement was better for PET/CT than for CT alone.[48] Risum and colleagues[49] prospectively compared PET/CT, US, and CT for detecting recurrent ovarian cancer in 60 patients with 68 studies. The inclusion criteria were remission of 3 months or more and recurrence suspected from physical examination, US, or increasing CA-125 level (>50 U/mL or >15% more than baseline level). The sensitivities of US, CT, and PET/CT for diagnosing recurrence were 66% (P = .003), 81% (P = .0001), and 97% (P<.0001), respectively with 90% specificity. Multiple recurrent tumors were found using PET/CT in 27 (69%) of 39 patients with solitary tumors on US and in 8 (42%) of 19 patients with solitary tumors on CT. The investigators concluded that the diagnostic value of PET/CT for detecting recurrent ovarian cancer was higher than those of US and CT and that PET/CT more accurately identified patients with solitary recurrence.[49]

Serum CA-125 levels are often used to follow patients who have ovarian cancer and to suggest recurrence. Sheng and colleagues[50] reported the PET/CT findings on 26 patients with rising CA-125 levels (doubling or greater in 2 months), with 14/17 greater than 35 kU/L, most associated with a negative CT scan. In nearly all patients, PET was able to detect recurrent tumor, although more foci appeared to be detected by PET in patients with higher CA-125 levels.[50] Thus, it is common to have a negative or equivocal CT and a positive PET scan if serum markers are increased or increasing. An example of FDG-PET/CT scans obtained in the setting of suspected recurrence with rising CA-125 levels is shown in **Fig. 1**.

Several of the authors of this review have begun to evaluate the comparative performance of PET/CT versus CA-125 in the setting of possible recurrence of ovarian carcinoma.

Javadi and colleagues[51] recently gave a preliminary report on the relative performance of PET/CT versus CA-125 levels in a group of 17 patients with histologically proven stage III/IV ovarian cancer

and concurrently increased CA-125 at the time of primary diagnosis who were suspected of tumor recurrence, analyzing 86 FDG-PET/CT scans with concurrent CA-125 measurements. Indications for PET/CT included patients assessed for treatment response and patients with suspected recurrent disease. FDG-PET/CT positivity was determined from the clinical report. The Gynecologic Cancer Intergroup defines CA-125 to be positive for progression when CA-125 is twice the upper limit of normal (35 U/mL) for patients who have normalized CA-125 after therapy, and CA-125 of twice the nadir value if the levels did not normalize. The sensitivity of FDG-PET/CT was 86%, much higher than the 17% seen for CA-125 levels using the GIG 35 U/mL cut off. Specificity was 86% for FDG-PET/CT, although it was 100% for CA-125 level increases. Examples of the relationship between PET/CT positivity and CA-125 levels are shown in **Figs. 1** and **2**. These data are similar to those recently reported by Pan and colleagues[52] in a study of 26 women, in which FDG-PET/CT had a sensitivity of 100% with a specificity of 85%, and, by contrast, CA-125 level increase was 58% sensitive but 100% specific. Other serum markers, such as carcinoembryonic antigen, were fairly specific but had poor sensitivity. Thus, a substantial fraction of women with ovarian cancer recurrence have negative CA-125 levels.[52]

A prospective multicenter study in Australia assessed the incremental information provided by and the effect of FDG-PET/CT on the management of 90 women with suspected recurrent ovarian cancer (restaging) based on increased CA-125, anatomic imaging, or clinical symptoms.[53] Referring doctors were asked to specify a pre-PET management plan, whether management was altered after PET/CT, and the effect (rated as none, low, medium, high) of PET/CT on patient management. Patients were followed at 6 and 12 months and clinical status, evidence of recurrence, and progression were recorded. PET/CT identified at least 168 additional sites of disease in 61 patients (68%), not identified by conventional imaging. PET/CT affected management in 60% of patients (49% high, 11% medium effect). Patients in whom more disease was detected with PET/CT were more likely to progress in the following 12 months. The investigators concluded that, for women with previously treated ovarian carcinoma with suspected recurrent disease, PET/CT was superior in the detection of nodal, peritoneal, and subcapsular liver disease and that the data supported replacing CT with PET/CT in this setting.[53] Thus, this

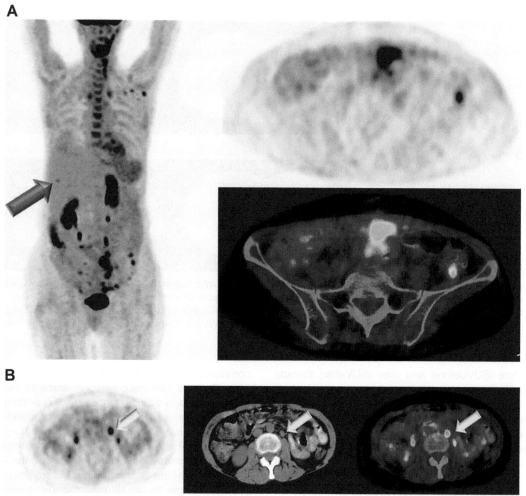

Fig. 1. (A) True-positive FDG-PET/CT and increased CA-125 in recurrent ovarian cancer. A woman with markedly increased CA-125 level at 176 U/mL was referred to FDG-PET/CT for suspected recurrence. PET/CT demonstrates new peritoneal implants (transverse image, *right bottom*), lymph node metastases, and a liver surface implant (*arrow* on maximum intensity projection). (B) True-positive FDG-PET/CT and false-negative CA-125 in recurrent ovarian cancer. A woman with ovarian cancer was referred for FDG-PET/CT because of unclear clinical complaints. Concurrent CA-125 levels were normal at 18 U/mL. Transaxial FDG-PET (*left*) and CT (*right*) images showed a left-sided FDG-avid paraaortic lymph node (*arrow*). Biopsy of node confirmed ovarian carcinoma.

prospective trial was highly supportive of prior smaller prospective, and of retrospective, trials.

FDG IMAGING MONITORING RESPONSE OF OVARIAN CANCER TO THERAPY

There is increased use of PET/CT for evaluating response to neoadjuvant, adjuvant, or standard chemotherapy, or radiotherapy but the literature is just evolving and studies are small. In a prospective study of 33 patients with advanced-stage ovarian cancer (FIGO stage IIIC and IV) receiving neoadjuvant chemotherapy before cytoreductive surgery, FDG-PET of the abdomen and pelvis was obtained before treatment and after the first and third cycles of chemotherapy. A significant correlation was observed between FDG-PET metabolic response after the first (threshold of 20% decline in standardized uptake value [SUV]) and third cycle of chemotherapy (threshold of 55% decline in SUV) and overall survival. The investigators concluded that FDG-PET seems to be a promising tool for early prediction of response to chemotherapy.[54] In another study of 21 patients with advanced gynecologic malignancies (including 8 patients with ovarian cancer) receiving FDG-PET examinations before and after completion of chemotherapy or chemoradiotherapy, Nishiyama and colleagues[55] applied semiquantitative SUV analysis at the primary tumor for both

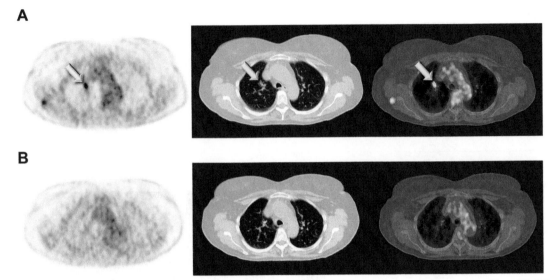

Fig. 2. False-positive PET and true-negative CA-125. (*A*) A patient with suspected ovarian cancer and low CA-125 levels at 6 U/mL underwent FDG-PET/CT, which indicated the presence of an FDG-avid pulmonary nodule (*arrow*) suspicious for metastasis of ovarian cancer. (*B*) Follow-up FDG-PET/CT showed that the abnormal tracer activity in the lung had resolved on PET (*left*) without antineoplastic treatment. Concurrent CA-125 level remained at normal levels at 8 U/mL.

before (SUVbefore) and after (SUVafter) therapy respectively, and determined its percent decline. Based on histopathologic analysis of the specimens obtained at surgery, patients were classified as responders or nonresponders. SUVafter in 10 responders was significantly lower than in the 11 nonresponders (*P*<.005). Using an SUVafter of 3.8 as the cutoff for differentiating between responders and nonresponders, FDG-PET showed a sensitivity of 90%, a specificity of 63.6%, and an accuracy of 76.2%. The percent change value in the responders was significantly higher than that in the nonresponders (*P*<.0005). Taking a percent change of 65 as the cutoff, FDG-PET showed a sensitivity of 90%, a specificity of 81.8%, and an accuracy of 85.7% for differentiating between responders and nonresponders.[55]

FDG IMAGING SURVEILLANCE OF OVARIAN CANCER

True prospective systematic surveillance studies evaluating tumor recurrence in patients who are clinically disease free and not on specific therapies have not been reported so far in ovarian cancer. Most of the studies have been retrospective and were performed at varying points in the disease management algorithm. Thus, the precise role of PET/CT in surveillance is still evolving (**Table 2**). The study of Rose and colleagues[56] could possibly be viewed as restaging or as surveillance, because it involved an assessment after therapy was

completed. FDG-PET results were correlated with findings on SLL in 22 patients with advanced-stage ovarian cancer (n = 17) or peritoneal carcinoma (N = 5) who had achieved complete clinical remission and had normal CA-125 level after 6 cycles of chemotherapy Persistent disease was found in 13 of the 22 patients (59%) on SLL including 1.5 cm macroscopic disease (n = 1), macroscopic disease less than 1 cm (n = 8), and microscopic disease (n = 4). PET only detected the 1.5 cm macroscopic disease and 1 of the sites with microscopic disease. The 10% sensitivity for all lesions is associated with a 100% sensitivity for lesions more than 1 cm in diameter, similar to that of Bristow and colleagues[45] Thus, PET has consistently performed well for macroscopic disease, but commonly fails in low tumor volume disease.

In a retrospective chart review, Thrall and colleagues[57] identified 59 FDG-PET/CT scans with intravenous contrast (in 39 patients with ovarian cancer) performed for restaging (47 scans), monitoring response to treatment (8 scans), or surveillance (4 scans). Four patients were scanned in lieu of SLL and all were negative with no recurrent disease detected during a follow-up period of 6 months. Garcia-Velloso and colleagues[58] retrospectively evaluated the diagnostic yield of FDG-PET for the diagnosis of recurrent ovarian cancer. Eighty FDG-PET scans were performed on 55 patients owing to suspicion of relapse (restaging), and 45 FDG-PET scans were

Table 2
Performance of FDG imaging in surveillance of patients with ovarian cancer

Author	N	Sensitivity (%)	Specificity (%)	Standard of Reference
Rose et al[56]	22 (17 ovary)	10	42	SLL
Zimny et al[38]	48	65	86	Histology/follow-up of median 22 mo
Nakamoto et al[39]	12	67	89	Histopathology/$\geq$6 mo clinical follow-up

performed on 31 patients who were clinically disease free (surveillance). In the patients who underwent imaging for surveillance the sensitivity, specificity, PPV, NPV, and accuracy were 55%, 88%, 78%, 71%, and 73% respectively. Thus, PET can perform well in a surveillance setting, but more systematic study is essential to fully define the role of the method in this setting, when it should be done, and whether it changes outcomes.

FDG IMAGING FOR PROGNOSIS OF PATIENTS WHO HAVE OVARIAN CANCER

Determining prognosis at any of several times including after cytoreductive surgery, adjuvant chemotherapy, or at presentation before any therapy has been assessed by Kim and colleagues.[59] They retrospectively compared the prognostic value of FDG-PET with SLL in 55 patients with advanced ovarian cancer who had undergone cytoreductive surgery and adjuvant chemotherapy.[59] Thirty patients underwent SLL and 25 patients underwent FDG-PET. Disease-free interval (40.5 ± 11.6 months and 48.6 ± 12.1 months respectively in the PET and SLL groups) and progression-free interval (28.8 ± 12.7 months and 30.6 ± 13.7 months respectively in the PET and SLL groups) were similar and the investigators concluded that FDG-PET could be used as a substitute for SLL in the follow-up of patients with ovarian cancer. Avril and colleagues[54] showed a better prognosis in patients who have a brisk decline in SUV to chemotherapy than was seen in the nonresponding groups. Cho and colleagues[60] retrospectively assessed the correlation of PET positivity with tumor recurrence and vascularity, Ki-67, p53, and histologic grade in 19 patients with recurrent ovarian cancer before SLL. FDG avidity revealed positive correlations with microvessel density and mitotic activity. Thus, it seems biologically reasonable to expect that declines in tumor metabolic activity would likely be linked to relevant biologic changes. The issue of stage migration with PET has been addressed recently. With the superior sensitivity of PET for stage IV disease, more patients with small-volume stage IV disease are being identified. This finding may result in improved survival for patients with stage III and IV disease, although a smaller fraction of patients will have stage III disease.[36]

FDG IMAGING–BASED CHANGES IN MANAGEMENT OF OVARIAN CANCER

Simcock and colleagues[61] prospectively evaluated the effect of PET/CT in the management of recurrent epithelial ovarian cancer. PET/CT results showed a disease distribution that was different from the known (pre-PET/CT) distribution in 64% of scans. PET/CT showed less disease than known in 9% and more disease in 52% of scans. PET/CT resulted in a substantial management change in 58% of patients. The investigators concluded that PET/CT modifies the assessment of the distribution of recurrent ovarian cancer, alters patient management in a substantial proportion of patients, and seems to offer prognostic information.

Another report showed that PET seemed to induce an intermodality change in management in 62.8% of patients with suspected recurrent ovarian carcinoma.[62] Mangili and colleagues[63] compared PET/CT with CT in 32 patients. Intermodality changes in management after PET/CT examinations were indicated in 14/32 (44%) patients in the chart review. The most common management change was from observation to chemotherapy. The prospective study by Fulham[53] also showed an approximately 60% change in management versus standard imaging results. The large National Oncologic PET Registry in the United States included more than 3000 patients with ovarian or uterine cancers.[64] In both the staging/restaging and the treatment monitoring groups, changes in management of 30% to 40% of patients were observed following PET imaging. Although identifying precise changes in ovarian cancer management is challenging, these data are supportive of a significant fraction of the PET scans resulting in major management changes.

Economic analyses of PET are limited. In one model, PET reduced the number of laparotomies for diagnosis, from70% to just 5%, with estimated cost savings ranging between $2000 and $12,000/case as a result of avoidance of many surgical procedures.[65] A recent economic analysis retrospectively evaluated 32 patients with suspected ovarian cancer recurrence, studied by both contrast-enhanced abdominal CT and PET/CT. Three different diagnostic strategies were evaluated and compared[1]: CT only, or baseline strategy[2]; PET/CT for negative CT, or strategy A[3]; PET/CT for all, or strategy B.[66] Expected costs, avoided surgery, and incremental cost-effectiveness ratio (ICER) were calculated for each strategy to identify which was the most cost-effective. The number of positive patients increased from baseline strategy (20/32) to strategies A and B (30/32 and 29/32 respectively). PET/CT reoriented physician choice in 31% and 62% of patients (strategies A and B respectively). Strategy A is dominated by strategy B, which is more expensive (2909 euro vs 2958 euro) but also more effective (3 cases of surgery avoided) and presents an ICER of 226.77 euro per surgery avoided (range 49.50–433.00 euro).[66] Introduction of PET/CT in this population was therefore cost-effective and allowed redirection of the clinical management of patients toward more appropriate therapeutic choices. These data therefore support the initial use of PET/CT in evaluating ovarian cancer recurrence.

FDG-PET/MR IMAGING IN OVARIAN CANCER

PET/CT is the established hybrid imaging method for ovarian carcinoma, but combinations of PET and MR imaging are being explored and this technology is evolving rapidly. The combination of PET and MR imaging using software fusion techniques has been examined by Nakajo and colleagues[67] in 31 patients with ovarian cancer. The investigators concluded that anatomic localization was superior for PET-MR imaging fusion than for PET/CT. However, diagnostic accuracy was not formally evaluated. Nonetheless, although PET/MR imaging could play a growing role in ovarian cancer imaging in the future, it is still in its infancy.

SUMMARY

PET/CT imaging of ovarian carcinoma is increasingly accepted and disseminated into clinical practice. Currently, there is not an established role for PET imaging in screening for ovarian cancer. It is also not clear that the performance of PET/CT is adequate to characterize ovarian masses as malignant or benign because some false negatives are seen in borderline disease and in those tumors with substantial cystic components. Recent results with PET/CT have been encouraging. The high sensitivity in detecting ovarian cancers could lead to delays or avoidance of surgery in the PET-negative group or to laparoscopic approaches as opposed to surgery. However, missing ovarian cancer would not be acceptable. There seem to be sufficient data showing less than optimal sensitivity. Therefore, an approach using FDG-PET/CT to make the determination as to whether a mass requires surgery cannot be confidently recommended. In postmenopausal women, intense FDG uptake in an ovarian mass is highly concerning for ovarian cancer. Such a finding can be seen incidentally in a busy PET/CT practice, because of the prevalence of ovarian cancer in the cancer population, and warrants further investigation. More data, including careful prospective trials in adequate numbers of patients using state of the art PET/CT, are required before PET/CT could be adopted as a tool to make triage decisions regarding ovarian masses.

Substantial data now exist to show PET/CT to be consistently superior to CT alone in the detection of recurrent ovarian cancer for most histologies. Although prospective studies showing survival benefit in patients imaged with PET would be desirable, they are unlikely to be forthcoming, especially given the increasing clinical acceptance of PET/CT in patient management. Although many studies are retrospective, most have shown the limited ability of FDG imaging to detect disease recurrence of lesions less than 5 to 10 mm in maximum diameter.

The most established indication for PET/CT seems to be in patients with clinical suspicion of recurrent ovarian carcinoma based on rising CA-125 levels (more than 35 U/mL or doubling of the nadir achieved after primary treatment) and negative or equivocal morphologic imaging findings. However, a significant number of patients with ovarian carcinoma recur with CA-125 levels less than 35 U/mL, raising the possibility of PET surveillance for recurrence in high-risk groups. Given the rapidly growing acceptance of PET/CT, it is increasingly common, despite a limited number of studies, to use PET/CT instead of CT alone in the imaging management of ovarian cancer, for treatment response assessment as well as for follow-up. The roles of FDG imaging in ovarian cancer treatment response assessment are less well explored, but initial data are consistent with those of other solid tumors (ie, brisk declines in glycolysis are associated with better responses and prognosis). The role of FDG-PET/CT in surveillance remains under evaluation, but it is increasingly applied if there are reasonable therapeutic alternatives for patients. In summary, FDG-PET/CT is now a standard tool in imaging women with ovarian carcinoma at multiple phases of the disease.

REFERENCES

1. Cancer facts and figures. Atlanta (GA): American Cancer Society; 2009. Available at: http://www.cancer.org.
2. Mourits MJ, de Bock GH. Managing hereditary ovarian cancer. Maturitas 2009;64(3):172–6.
3. Kauff ND, Barakat RR. Risk-reducing salpingo-oophorectomy in patients with germline mutations in BRCA1 or BRCA2. J Clin Oncol 2007;25:2921–7.
4. Bhoola S, Hoskins W. Diagnosis and management of epithelial ovarian cancer. Obstet Gynecol 2006;107:1399–410.
5. Jacobs I, Stabile I, Bridges J, et al. Multimodal approach to screening for ovarian cancer. Lancet 1988;1:268–71.
6. Jacobs I, Davies AP, Bridges J, et al. Prevalence screening for ovarian cancer in postmenopausal women by CA 125 measurement and ultrasonography. BMJ 1993;306:1030–4.
7. Jacobs IJ, Skates SJ, MacDonald N, et al. Screening for ovarian cancer: a pilot randomised controlled trial. Lancet 1999;353:1207–10.
8. Skates SJ, Menon U, MacDonald N, et al. Calculation of the risk of ovarian cancer from serial CA-125 values for preclinical detection in postmenopausal women. J Clin Oncol 2003;21(Suppl 10):206–10.
9. Buys SS, Partridge E, Greene MH, et al. Ovarian cancer screening in the Prostate, Lung, Colorectal and Ovarian (PLCO) cancer screening trial: findings from the initial screen of a randomized trial. Am J Obstet Gynecol 2005;193:1630–9.
10. Menon U, Skates SJ, Lewis S, et al. Prospective study using the risk of ovarian cancer algorithm to screen for ovarian cancer. J Clin Oncol 2005;23:7919–26.
11. Liu J, Xu Y, Wang J. Ultrasonography, computed tomography and magnetic resonance imaging for diagnosis of ovarian carcinoma. Eur J Radiol 2007;62:328–34.
12. American College of Obstetricians and Gynecologists, ACOG Committee on Practice Bulletins—Gynecology, ACOG Committee on Genetics, et al. ACOG Practice Bulletin No. 103: hereditary breast and ovarian cancer syndrome. Obstet Gynecol 2009;113:957–66.
13. Gadducci A, Cosio S, Zola P, et al. Surveillance procedures for patients treated for epithelial ovarian cancer: a review of the literature. Int J Gynecol Cancer 2007;17:21–31.
14. Qayyum A, Coakley FV, Westphalen AC, et al. Role of CT and MR imaging in predicting optimal cytoreduction of newly diagnosed primary epithelial ovarian cancer. Gynecol Oncol 2005;96:301–6.
15. Hess LM, Benham-Hutchins M, Herzog TJ, et al. A meta-analysis of the efficacy of intra-peritoneal cisplatin for the front-line treatment of ovarian cancer. Int J Gynecol Cancer 2007;17:561–70.
16. Armstrong DK, Bundy B, Wenzel L, et al. Intraperitoneal cisplatin and paclitaxel in ovarian cancer. N Engl J Med 2006;354:34–43.
17. See HT, Kavanaugh JJ. The MD Anderson manual of medical oncology. Chapter 22, Ovarian Cancer. New York: McGraw-Hill; 2006. p. 543–78.
18. Wahl RL, Hutchins GD, Buchsbaum DJ, et al. 18F-2-deoxy-2-fluoro-D-glucose uptake into human tumor xenografts. Feasibility studies for cancer imaging with positron-emission tomography. Cancer 1991;67:1544–50.
19. Brown RS, Fisher SJ, Wahl RL. Autoradiographic evaluation of the intra-tumoral distribution of 2-deoxy-D-glucose and monoclonal antibodies in xenografts of human ovarian adenocarcinoma. J Nucl Med 1993;34:75–82.
20. Zhuang H, Pourdehnad M, Lambright ES, et al. Dual time point 18F-FDG PET imaging for differentiating malignant from inflammatory processes. J Nucl Med 2001;42:1412–7.
21. Shen YY, Chen LK, Liao AC, et al. Application of PET and PET/CT imaging for cancer screening. Anticancer Res 2004;24:4103–8.
22. Schöder H, Gönen M. Screening for cancer with PET and PET/CT: potential and limitations. J Nucl Med 2007;1(Suppl 48):4S–18S.
23. Lerman H, Metser U, Grisaru D, et al. Normal and abnormal F18-FDG endometrial and ovarian uptake in pre- and postmenopausal patients: assessment by PET/CT. J Nucl Med 2004;45:266–71.
24. Kim SK, Kang KW, Roh JW, et al. Incidental ovarian F18-FDG accumulation on PET: correlation with the menstrual cycle. Eur J Nucl Med Mol Imaging 2005;32:757–63.
25. Zhu ZH, Cheng WY, Cheng X, et al. [Characteristics of physiological uptake of uterus and ovaries on 18F-fluorodeoxyglucose positron emission tomography]. Zhongguo Yi Xue Ke Xue Yuan Xue Bao 2007;29:124–9 [in Chinese].
26. Togashi K. Ovarian cancer: the clinical role of US, CT and MRI. Eur Radiol 2003;13:L87–104.

27. Hubner KF, McDonald TW, Niethammer JG, et al. Assessment of primary and metastatic ovarian cancer by positron emission tomography (PET) using 2-[F18]deoxyglucose (2-[F18]FDG). Gynecol Oncol 1993;51:197–204.

28. Rieber A, Nussla K, Stohr I, et al. Preoperative diagnosis of ovarian tumors with MR imaging: comparison with transvaginal sonography, positron emission tomography and histologic findings. AJR Am J Roentgenol 2001;177:123–9.

29. Kawahara K, Yoshida Y, Kurokawa, et al. Evaluation of positron emission tomography with tracer 18-fluorodeoxyglucose in addition to magnetic resonance imaging in the diagnosis of ovarian cancer in selected women after ultrasonography. J Comput Assist Tomogr 2004;28:505–16.

30. Risum S, Hogdall C, Loft A, et al. The diagnostic value of PET/CT for primary ovarian cancer–a prospective study. Gynecol Oncol 2007;105: 145–9.

31. Nam EJ, Yun MJ, Oh YT, et al. Diagnosis and staging of primary ovarian cancer: correlation between PET/CT, Doppler US, and CT or MRI. Gynecol Oncol 2010;116:389–94.

32. Gjelsteen AC, Ching BH, Meyermann MW, et al. CT, MRI, PET, PET/CT, and ultrasound in the evaluation of obstetric and gynecologic patients. Surg Clin North Am 2008;88:361–90.

33. Yoshida Y, Kurokawa T, Kawahara K, et al. Incremental benefits of FDG positron emission tomography over CT alone for the preoperative staging of ovarian cancer. AJR Am J Roentgenol 2004;182: 227–33.

34. Turlakow A, Yeung HW, Salmon AS, et al. Peritoneal carcinomatosis: role of (18)F-FDG PET. J Nucl Med 2003;44:1407–12.

35. Kitajima K, Murakami K, Yamasaki E, et al. Diagnostic accuracy of integrated FDG-PET/contrast-enhanced CT in staging ovarian cancer: comparison with enhanced CT. Eur J Nucl Med Mol Imaging 2008;35:1912–20.

36. Risum S, Høgdall C, Loft A, et al. Does the use of diagnostic PET/CT cause stage migration in patients with primary advanced ovarian cancer? Gynecol Oncol 2010;116:395–8.

37. Yen RF, Sun SS, Shen YY, et al. Whole body positron emission tomography with 18F-fluoro-2-deoxyglucose for the detection of recurrent ovarian cancer. Anticancer Res 2001;21:3691–4.

38. Zimny M, Siggelkow W, Schroder W, et al. 2-[Fluorine-18]-fluoro-2-deoxy-D-glucose positron emission tomography in the diagnosis of recurrent ovarian cancer. Gynecol Oncol 2001;83:310–5.

39. Nakamoto Y, Saga T, Ishimori T, et al. Clinical value of positron emission tomography with FDG for recurrent ovarian cancer. AJR Am J Roentgenol 2001; 176:1449–54.

40. Torizuka T, Nobezawa S, Kanno T, et al. Ovarian cancer recurrence: role of whole-body positron emission tomography using 2-[fluorine-18]-fluoro-2-deoxy-D-glucose. Eur J Nucl Med Mol Imaging 2002;29:797–803.

41. Takekuma M, Maeda M, Ozawa T, et al. Positron emission tomography with 18F-fluoro-2-deoxyglucose for the detection of recurrent ovarian cancer. Int J Clin Oncol 2005;10:177–81.

42. Nanni C, Rubello D, Farsad M, et al. (18)F-FDG PET/CT in the evaluation of recurrent ovarian cancer: a prospective study on forty-one patients. Eur J Surg Oncol 2005;31:792–7.

43. Chung HH, Kang WJ, Kim JW, et al. Role of [18F] FDG PET/CT in the assessment of suspected recurrent ovarian cancer: correlation with clinical or histological findings. Eur J Nucl Med Mol Imaging 2007;34:480–6.

44. Bristow RE, del Carmen MG, Pannu HK, et al. Clinically occult recurrent ovarian cancer: patient selection for secondary cytoreductive surgery using combined PET/CT. Gynecol Oncol 2003;90: 519–28.

45. Bristow RE, Giuntoli RL 2nd, Pannu HK, et al. Combined PET/CT for detecting recurrent ovarian cancer limited to retroperitoneal lymph nodes. Gynecol Oncol 2005;99:294–300.

46. Pannu HK, Cohade C, Bristow RE, et al. PET-CT detection of abdominal recurrence of ovarian cancer: radiologic-surgical correlation. Abdom Imaging 2004;29:398–403.

47. Sironi S, Messa C, Mangili G, et al. Integrated FDG PET/CT in patients with persistent ovarian cancer: correlation with histologic findings. Radiology 2004;233:433–40.

48. Sebastian S, Lee SI, Horowitz NS, et al. PET-CT vs. CT alone in ovarian cancer recurrence. Abdom Imaging 2008;33:112–8.

49. Risum S, Høgdall C, Markova E, et al. Influence of 2-(18F) fluoro-2-deoxy-D-glucose positron emission tomography/computed tomography on recurrent ovarian cancer diagnosis and on selection of patients for secondary cytoreductive surgery. Int J Gynecol Cancer 2009;19:600–4.

50. Sheng XG, Zhang XL, Fu Z, et al. [Value of positron emission tomography-CT imaging combined with continual detection of CA125 in serum for diagnosis of early asymptomatic recurrence of epithelial ovarian carcinoma]. Zhonghua Fu Chan Ke Za Zhi 2007;42:460–3 [in Chinese].

51. Javadi M, Shruti A, Bristow R, et al. FDG-PET/CT in assessing ovarian cancer recurrence and patient outcome: comparison to CA-125. J Nucl Med 2009;50(Suppl 2):174.

52. Pan HS, Lee SL, Huang LW, et al. Combined positron emission tomography-computed tomography and tumor markers for detecting recurrent

ovarian cancer. Arch Gynecol Obstet 2010 Mar 11. DOI:10.1007/s00404-010-1404-6.

53. Fulham MJ, Carter J, Baldey A, et al. The impact of PET-CT in suspected recurrent ovarian cancer: a prospective multi-centre study as part of the Australian PET Data Collection Project. Gynecol Oncol 2009;112:462–8.

54. Avril N, Sassen S, Schmalfeldt B, et al. Prediction of response to neoadjuvant chemotherapy by sequential F-18-fluorodeoxyglucose positron emission tomography in patients with advanced-stage ovarian cancer. J Clin Oncol 2005;23:7445–53.

55. Nishiyama Y, Yamamoto Y, Kanenishi K, et al. Monitoring the neoadjuvant therapy response in gynecological cancer patients using FDG PET. Eur J Nucl Med Mol Imaging 2008;35:287–95.

56. Rose PG, Faulhaber P, Miraldi F, et al. Positive emission tomography for evaluating a complete clinical response in patients with ovarian or peritoneal carcinoma: correlation with second-look laparotomy. Gynecol Oncol 2001;82:17–21.

57. Thrall MM, DeLoia JA, Gallion H, et al. Clinical use of combined positron emission tomography and computed tomography (FDG-PET/CT) in recurrent ovarian cancer. Gynecol Oncol 2007;105:17–22.

58. Garcia-Velloso MJ, Jurado M, Ceamanos C, et al. Diagnostic accuracy of FDG PET in the follow-up of platinum-sensitive epithelial ovarian carcinoma. Eur J Nucl Med Mol Imaging 2007;34:1396–405.

59. Kim S, Chung JK, Kang SB, et al. [18F]FDG PET as a substitute for second-look laparotomy in patients with advanced ovarian carcinoma. Eur J Nucl Med Mol Imaging 2004;31:196–201.

60. Cho SM, Park YG, Lee JM, et al. 18F-fluorodeoxyglucose positron emission tomography in patients with

recurrent ovarian cancer: in comparison with vascularity, Ki-67, p53, and histologic grade. Eur Radiol 2007;17:409–17.

61. Simcock B, Neesham D, Quinn M, et al. The impact of PET/CT in the management of recurrent ovarian cancer. Gynecol Oncol 2006;103:271–6.

62. Ruiz-Hernandez G, Delgado-Bolton RC, Fernandez-Perez C, et al. Impact of positron emission tomography with FDG-PET in treatment of patients with suspected recurrent ovarian cancer. Rev Esp Med Nucl 2005;24:113–26.

63. Mangili G, Picchio M, Sironi S, et al. Integrated PET/CT as a first-line re-staging modality in patients with suspected recurrence of ovarian cancer. Eur J Nucl Med Mol Imaging 2007;34:658–66.

64. Hillner BE, Siegel BA, Shields AF, et al. The impact of positron emission tomography (PET) on expected management during cancer treatment: findings of the National Oncologic PET Registry. Cancer 2009;115:410–8.

65. Smith GT, Hubner KF, McDonald T, et al. Cost analysis of FDG PET for managing patients with ovarian cancer. Clin Positron Imaging 1999;2:63–70.

66. Mansueto M, Grimaldi A, Mangili G, et al. Positron emission tomography/computed tomography introduction in the clinical management of patients with suspected recurrence of ovarian cancer: a cost-effectiveness analysis. Eur J Cancer Care (Engl) 2009;18:612–9.

67. Nakajo K, Tatsumi M, Inoue A, et al. Diagnostic performance of fluorodeoxyglucose positron emission tomography/magnetic resonance imaging fusion images of gynecological malignant tumors: comparison with positron emission tomography/computed tomography. Jpn J Radiol 2010;28:95–100.

PET/CT Imaging in Gynecologic Malignancies Other than Ovarian and Cervical Cancer

Priya Bhosale, MD[a],*, Revathy Iyer, MD[a],
Anuja Jhingran, MD[b], Donald Podoloff, MD[c]

KEYWORDS

- PET • Vaginal cancer • Vulvar cancer • Endometrial cancer
- Uterine cancer

Recent advances in PET and combined PET/computed tomography (CT) has increased its usefulness in oncologic imaging. The ability of PET to detect malignancy relies on the metabolic activity of the tumors that incorporate the PET radiopharmaceutical. When combined with CT, accurate anatomic localization of the metabolic abnormality is also possible. Currently PET with fluorine 18 [^{18}F]fluorodeoxyglucose (FDG) is the most commonly used agent for the diagnosis and staging of gynecologic malignancies. Newer agents such as [16α-^{18}F]fluoro-17β-estradiol (FES), a radiolabeled compound of the most bioactive type of estrogen, are being evaluated for detection of tumors that may be characterized as estrogen receptor (ER)−positive.[1–4] ^{18}F-labeled radioactive isotopes decay by positron emission and their detection indicates the presence of metabolically active sites of potential malignant origin.

The usefulness of FDG-PET imaging for patients with gynecologic cancers relies on the presence of increased glucose metabolism by the tumors. FDG-PET is the most commonly used technique to stage and detect recurrence in patients with cervical cancer. Patients with ovarian cancer also benefit from the use of FDG-PET to detect recurrent disease. In other gynecologic malignancies such as endometrial cancer, uterine sarcomas, vulvar cancer, and vaginal cancers, the role of FDG-PET/CT is not as well defined.

IMAGING PROTOCOL

Patients must fast for at least 6 hours before FDG-PET/CT. Acquisition is usually performed at least 60 minutes after injection of intravenous contrast. The half-life of [^{18}F]FDG is 110 minutes. Because FDG is excreted though the gastrointestinal and urinary tracts, physiologic activity in normal bowel, kidneys, ureters, and urinary bladder can limit the interpretation of FDG imaging in gynecologic malignancies. Technical modifications such as intravenous hydration with concomitant diuresis, continuous bladder irrigation, mechanical bowel

The authors have nothing to disclose.

[a] Department of Diagnostic Radiology, University of Texas MD Anderson Cancer Center, 1515 Holcombe, Houston, TX 77030, USA
[b] Department of Radiation Oncology Treatment, University of Texas MD Anderson Cancer Center, 1515 Holcombe, Houston, TX 77030, USA
[c] Department of Nuclear Medicine, University of Texas MD Anderson Cancer Center, 1515 Holcombe, Houston, TX 77030, USA
* Corresponding author. Department of Diagnostic Radiology, The University of Texas MD Anderson Cancer Center, 1515 Holcombe, Box 368, Houston, TX 77030.
E-mail address: Priya.bhosale@mdanderson.org

PET Clin 5 (2010) 463–475
doi:10.1016/j.cpet.2010.07.005
1556-8598/10/$ − see front matter. Published by Elsevier Inc.

preparation, or insertion of a Foley catheter can be performed.

In premenopausal patients, normal endometrial and ovarian uptake of FDG changes cyclically with the menstrual cycle. Endometrial activity and activity in the uterine fibroids increases during the menstrual and ovulatory phases. Endometriomas and corpus luteal cysts in the ovaries may also be FDG avid.[5] In situations in which it is uncertain whether the FDG activity is physiologic, repeat imaging can be performed in the early follicular phase of the menstrual cycle. Delayed imaging at 3 hours after FDG injection can also be obtained but is of limited value for patients with endometrial cancer.[2] In postmenopausal woman, increased uterine and ovarian FDG uptake is usually associated with malignancy and is much less likely to indicate a benign process.

ENDOMETRIAL CANCER

Endometrial cancer is the most common invasive gynecologic malignancy. Each year 25 women per 100,000 are diagnosed with this disease. The most common histology is adenocarcinoma. Most women present with well-differentiated or moderately differentiated endometrioid histology, and the 5-year survival is 84%.[6] Other histologic subtypes such as grade III endometrioid carcinoma and serous and clear cell tumors have a 5-year overall survival of 60% to 80% and a high incidence of relapse.[7–9] Although endometrial cancer is a disease affecting mainly postmenopausal women, up to 25% of cases occur in premenopausal patients.[10] The main risk factor for endometrial cancer is increased unopposed estrogen, which is associated with menopause, low parity, obesity, anovulation, and polycystic ovarian syndrome. Patients with hereditary conditions such as Lynch syndrome are also at increased risk. Endometrial cancer is usually detected early in postmenopausal patients as they typically present with dysfunctional uterine bleeding, and therefore more than 70% of patients have stage I disease at presentation.[6] Surgery is the primary means of staging for endometrial cancer, mainly in patients with organ-confined disease.[11] The tumor typically spreads by invasion of the myometrium, into the cervix, or via the fallopian tubes to the ovaries, and subsequently by local invasion to other organs of the pelvis. As the depth of myometrial invasion increases, so does the likelihood of lymphovascular invasion, with subsequent lymphatic and hematogenous metastases. Peritoneal spread of disease may also be encountered. Adjuvant radiation and chemotherapy are used in patients with advanced inoperable or recurrent disease and

imaging can play a role in defining tumor extent in these patients.[11]

FDG-PET has little value in detecting early-stage disease, which, in most patients, is confined to the uterus and has a low chance of metastatic dissemination. Currently, however, as a result of the use of hormone replacement therapy, irregular vaginal bleeding in postmenopausal women may be overlooked and investigations may be delayed.[12] Magnetic resonance (MR) imaging is considered the most accurate imaging technique for preoperative assessment of endometrial cancer, particularly with regard to myometrial invasion. MR imaging and CT can be used to evaluate the extent of extrauterine disease and can provide crucial information for treatment planning.[13] CA-125 combined with CT and MR imaging can further define the extrauterine spread of the tumor.[14,15]

Endometrial cancers can be estrogen sensitive and ER expression coupled with glucose metabolism using FES-PET/CT and FDG-PET/CT can be used to differentiate benign from malignant uterine tumors.[16] A recent study suggests that as the glucose metabolism in malignant endometrial lesions increases, the estrogen dependency decreases. This correlates with a progression from a lower to a higher risk of malignancy. A calculated FDG-PET to FES-PET ratio of 3.6 ± 2.1 in this study indicated high-risk cancer, compared with 1.3 ± 0.5 ($P<.01$) reported for low-risk malignancy; in endometrial hyperplasia the ratio was 0.3 ± 0.1 ($P<.005$). The study concludes that the FDG/FES ratio may be useful in the differential diagnosis of endometrial hyperplasia from endometrial cancer and for deciding on the appropriate therapeutic strategies for patients with malignant tumors.[17] Although FDG-PET/CT is of limited usefulness in the diagnosis of endometrial cancer,[5,18] it may have some added value in the diagnosis of extraabdominal disease and specifically in determining the extent of pelvic involvement, especially in the posttherapy surveillance of patients.

The reported maximum standard uptake value (SUV_{max}) measured in malignant endometrial lesions ranges from 2.3 to 8.2.[5] However, SUV_{max} measured in cases with physiologic tracer activity is also variable and ranges between 2.3 and 16.6 during the menstrual phase, between 1.1 and 5.7 during the proliferative phase, between 2 and 5.4 during the ovulatory phase, and between 1.3 and 5.6 during the secretory phase. Because of this wide range of values, diagnosis of malignancy cannot be based on SUV_{max} measurements only.[5] Furthermore, other processes such as endometrial hyperplasia, polyps, adenomyosis, leiomyoma, endometriosis, and endometrioma can also show metabolic activity.[19,20]

The presence and extent of extrauterine disease affects the rate of recurrence and overall survival. Staging of endometrial cancer according to the International Federation of Gynecology and Obstetrics (FIGO) surgical system consists of exploratory laparotomy, total abdominal hysterectomy, bilateral salpingo-oophorectomy, peritoneal lavage. and lymphadenectomy (Table 1). Clinical staging has been shown to result in understaging of 13% to 22% of patients with endometrial cancer and therefore imaging may assist in planning the optimal course of treatment in a significant number of cases.[2,21,22] The current recommendations based on FIGO staging (2009)[23] suggest that lymphadenectomy should be performed in patients with high-risk stage I disease and in patients with poor-prognosis histologic types such as serous or clear cell cancer, to determine whether these patients need adjuvant chemotherapy.

FDG imaging can be used in the preoperative setting to evaluate patients with endometrial carcinoma (Fig. 1).[2] FDG-PET had an overall higher specificity (100%) than CT/MR imaging (85.7%). The sensitivity of FDG-PET for detection of extrauterine lesions (excluding metastatic retroperitoneal lymph nodes) was 83.3% versus 66.7% for CT/MRI.[24]

In a recent study, overall lesion-based sensitivity, specificity, and accuracy of FDG-PET/CT for detecting nodal metastases were 53.3%, 99.6%, and 97.8%, respectively.[25] The sensitivity for detecting metastatic lesions varied with size. For lesions 4 mm or less in diameter the sensitivity was low at 16.7%, and increased to 66.7% for lesions between 5 and 9 mm.[26] An additional study indicated that the sensitivity of FDG-PET for detection of lymph node metastases smaller than 6 mm in size was poor. Therefore a negative FDG-PET should not preclude lymph node dissection.[2,24] FDG-PET/CT had a moderate sensitivity of 66% and high specificity of 95% for detection of lymph node metastases in patients with high-risk endometrial cancer. It also had a negative predictive value (NPV) of 98%, suggesting that FDG-PET/CT can be used to select patients who might benefit from lymphadenectomy and thereby prevent unnecessary perioperative complications in patients who would not benefit from a surgical procedure. FDG-PET/CT can also be helpful in assessing the extent of disease in patients who have undergone hysterectomy with incomplete operative staging.

Reports have shown that early detection of recurrent endometrial cancer with prompt initiation of therapy affects survival.[27,28] Serum tumor markers have been used in posttherapy follow-up of patients, although benign gynecologic conditions and nonmalignant processes can result in falsely increased values. True-positive increased markers do not indicate the site of

Table 1
FIGO staging of endometrial cancer

FIGO Staging	Current FIGO Classification	Treatment
Stage IA	Tumor limited to the endometrium	TAH with BSO ± surgical staging
Stage IB	Invasion to less than half of the myometrium	
Stage IC	Invasion equal to or more than half of the myometrium	
Stage IIA	Endocervical glandular involvement only	
Stage IIB	Cervical stromal invasion	Simple or radical hysterectomy ± radiation therapy
Stage IIIA	Tumor invades the serosa of the corpus uteri and/or adnexae and/or positive cytologic findings	
Stage IIIB	Vaginal metastases	TAH with BSO + radiation
Stage IIIC	Metastases to pelvic and/or paraaortic lymph nodes	
Stage IVA	Tumor invasion of bladder and/or bowel mucosa	
Stage IVB	Distant metastases, including intraabdominal metastasis and/or inguinal lymph nodes	TAH with BSO, radiation, and chemotherapy or hormone therapy

Abbreviations: BSO, bilateral salpingo-oophorectomy; TAH, total abdominal hysterectomy.

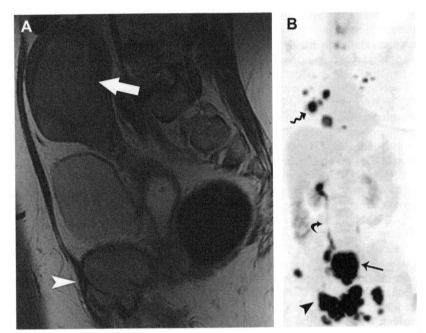

Fig. 1. A 65-year-old woman with endometrial cancer presented with low back pain. (*A*) Sagittal T2-weighted sequence through the pelvis shows a mass in the endometrium (*arrow*) and a metastasis to the pubis (*arrowhead*). (*B*) Coronal FDG-PET maximum intensity projection (MIP) image shows a mass in the endometrium (*arrow*) with right ureter obstruction (*curved arrow*), and multiple metastases to pelvic bones (*arrowhead*) and lungs (*squiggly arrow*).

recurrence.[29] Posttherapeutic changes can be difficult to differentiate from recurrent disease on CT, as they can have a similar morphologic appearance. Viable tumor is more likely to demonstrate hypermetabolism and thus FDG-PET/CT can differentiate recurrent malignancy from posttherapeutic changes. FDG imaging can detect both recurrence in the pelvis as well as metastatic spread in extrapelvic locations such as the lungs and abdomen in asymptomatic patients.[19,26] FDG-PET/CT has been used for postoperative evaluation of patients with suspected recurrence with sensitivity, specificity, and diagnostic accuracy ranging between 96% and 100%, between 78% and 88%, and between 90% and 93%, respectively. The positive predictive value (PPV) and NPV were 89% and 91%, respectively.[2,19,30] When FDG-PET was correlated with the information obtained from anatomic imaging modalities such as CT and MR imaging, the sensitivity was 100.0%, specificity was 88.2%, and accuracy was 93.3%.[30] FDG-PET/CT has also been evaluated in patients with endometrial cancer. In the setting of suspected recurrent disease, FDG-PET/CT has a reported sensitivity of 90% to 93%, a specificity of 81% to 100%, accuracy 87% to 96%, PPV 93% to 95%, and NPV of 100%.[26,31–33] FDG-PET/CT detected recurrent disease in patients with increased tumor markers

and negative CT and resulted in a change in clinical management in 21.9% of 64 patients.[32]

Local recurrence of endometrial cancer usually occurs at the vaginal apex, and patients may present with vaginal spotting. The 5-year cure rate in these patients is about 40% to 60%. FDG imaging can be used in these patients to exclude extrapelvic recurrence. Subsequent radiation treatment to the vaginal apex in patients with localized recurrence is reported to increase the cure rate to 90%.[34] FDG-PET/CT can result in additional changes in patient management such as initiation of unplanned therapy, changes to the treatment plan, and preclusion of planned procedures.[31] A negative FDG-PET/CT study in patients with treated endometrial cancer predicts significantly better progression-free survival than a positive result.[31]

UTERINE SARCOMAS

Uterine sarcomas are a group of rare and usually aggressive soft tissue malignancies representing less than 8% of uterine cancers.[35] They are more common in nonwhite women[35] and have a wide range of histologic appearances, from myomatous to osteous or stromal. There are 3 main subtypes of uterine sarcomas: carcinosarcoma, leiomyosarcoma, and endometrial stromal sarcoma.

Leiomyosarcomas resemble leiomyomas. Most patients are diagnosed between the sixth and seventh decade of life and present with abnormal uterine bleeding or a pelvic mass that may be confused with leiomyoma. The age-adjusted incidence rate is less than or equal to 35 per 100,000.[35] Staging of uterine sarcomas is similar to that for endometrial cancer and uses the FIGO system (see **Table 1**). Patients with disease clinically confined to the uterus (stage I or II) are frequently found to have unexpected spread at the time of surgery, typically hematogenous metastases to the lungs. About 50% of patients have disease recurrence.[36–39] Thorough knowledge of tumor pathway dissemination is necessary as sometimes other malignancies can be seen in conjunction with primary uterine neoplasms. These should not be mistaken for metastases and a biopsy should be performed for confirmation (**Fig. 2**) so that appropriate therapy can be instated.

There is no standardized preoperative imaging for uterine sarcoma. The current literature suggests that CT is commonly used.[40,41] The use of FDG-PET is not well defined for these tumors although they demonstrate FDG uptake.[42] In the preoperative setting, FDG-PET identifies distant metastases and can prevent futile attempts at

curative surgery.[43] Umesaki and colleagues[43] reported that FDG-PET detected leiomyosarcoma with an accuracy of 100% in a small study of 5 patients, compared with an accuracy of 80% for MR imaging. However, FDG-PET was unable to detect metastases in subcentimeter lymph nodes. Because of their aggressive tumor biology, leiomyosarcoma typically recurs within 2 years of initial treatment.[38,44] Lactate dehydrogenase (LDH) and CA-125 are the tumor markers generally used to follow these patients. Cross-sectional imaging modalities such as CT and MR imaging can be impaired for detection of recurrence in the presence of acute edema and fibrosis after treatment leading to delay in diagnosis and further treatment.[45,46]

The sensitivity to chemotherapy or radiation therapy differs between the 3 subtypes of uterine sarcomas. Radiotherapy is more beneficial for local control of carcinosarcoma but does not seem to improve survival, whereas leiomyosarcomas are chemosensitive.[47,48] There is no role for adjuvant chemotherapy in these patients, and close surveillance is necessary to detect relapse so that therapy can be reinstated.[47]

Compared with CT, FDG-PET had a better detection rate for extrapelvic recurrence. The

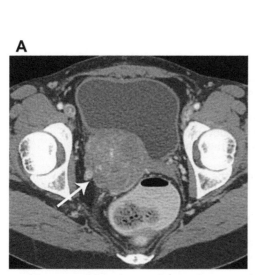
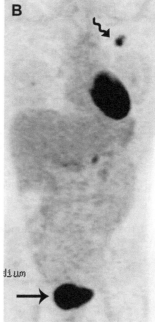

Fig. 2. A 47-year-old woman with endometrial stromal sarcoma. (*A*) Axial contrast-enhanced CT scan of the pelvis shows an enhancing mass consistent with the primary tumor (*arrow*). (*B*) Coronal FDG-PET MIP image shows a large hypermetabolic mass in the pelvis consistent with the known endometrial sarcoma (*arrow*) and an additional FDG-avid focus in the left lung (*squiggly arrow*). At biopsy the lung lesion was diagnosed as a second primary lung cancer.

sensitivity of FDG-PET was 100% compared with 85.7% for CT.[49,50] In another study of 36 patients, FDG-PET or PET/CT had a sensitivity, specificity, accuracy, PPV, and NPV of 92.9%, 100%, 94.4%, 100%, and 80%, respectively, in symptomatic patients. In asymptomatic patients with suspected recurrence, these values were 87.5%, 95.5%, 93.3%, 87.5%, and 95.5%, respectively.[51] Despite the ability to detect recurrence, FDG-PET did not improve overall survival.[43]

VAGINAL CANCER

Vaginal cancer is predominantly diagnosed in older women, starting as a rule in the seventh decade of life, and accounts for less than 3% of gynecologic malignancies.[52,53] In the United States, there are less than 2500 new cases and 800 deaths annually.[7] The most common histologic type is squamous cell carcinoma, which accounts for nearly 80% of all cases.[53] The factors that increase the patient's lifetime risk are early coitarche, multiple sexual partners, smoking, diethylstilbestrol exposure in utero,[54,55] and human papillomavirus (HPV) infection.[56] Bleeding is an associated symptom and is always present in patients with advanced disease. These tumors can be located throughout the vagina and are uni- or multifocal. Vaginal malignancy is usually diagnosed with Pap smear. Clinical staging is based on the FIGO system (Table 2).[23] Tumor spread is typically by local invasion, lymphatic dissemination to inguinal and pelvic lymph nodes, and hematogenous spread to the lungs. The lymph node drainage pattern differs depending on the location of tumor. For example, tumors in the upper third of the vagina drain into the pelvic lymph nodes, internal and external iliac chain, and obturator nodes, whereas tumors from the lower third drain into deep pelvic lymph nodes, femoral, and inguinal nodes.[57] Local excision is performed if the lesion is noninvasive and confined to one area. Invasive carcinoma involves the upper third of the vagina in more than half of the cases. MR imaging and CT have been used for staging vaginal cancer and to identify metastatic lesions. In early-stage disease, radiation therapy or radical surgery can be curative (Fig. 3).[52]

The reported 5-year survival for stage I disease is approximately 75% and in advanced disease it drops to 50%.[52] In our center, the 5-year disease-specific survival is 85% for stage I, 78% for stage II, and 58% for stages III and IV.[58] Adenocarcinoma has low survival rates of approximately 34% versus 58% for squamous cell cancers ($P<.01$). Among patients treated with radiation therapy alone, adenocarcinoma has a much higher rate of distant metastases compared with squamous cell tumors.[59]

Lamoreaux and colleagues[60] compared the results of CT with FDG-PET imaging in 23 patients with stage II and IV vaginal carcinoma and found that FDG-PET identified all metabolically active primary tumors for a sensitivity of 100%, and detected metastatic lymph nodes in 35% of patients compared with 17% by CT. The FIGO staging based on clinical examination does not incorporate adenopathy into the staging system. Thus

Table 2
FIGO staging of primary vaginal cancer

FIGO Staging	Current FIGO Classification	Treatment
Stage 0	Carcinoma in situ; vaginal intraepithelial neoplasia grade III	Radical surgery or radiation to the primary lesion
Stage I	The carcinoma is limited to the vaginal wall	
Stage II	The carcinoma has involved the subvaginal tissue but has not extended to the pelvic wall	
Stage III	The carcinoma has extended to the pelvic wall or suspicious pelvic/inguinal lymph nodes are present	Radiation to primary with adjuvant radiation to the metastases and/or chemotherapy
Stage IV	The tumor has extended beyond the true pelvis or has involved the mucosa of the bladder or rectum; bullous edema as such does not permit a case to be allotted to stage IV	
Stage IVA	Tumor invades bladder and/or rectal mucosa and/or direct extension beyond the true pelvis	
Stage IVB	Spread to distant organs	

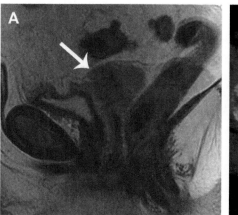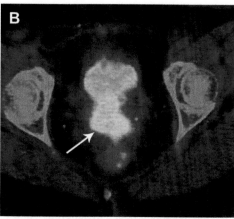

Fig. 3. A 68-year-old woman with postmenopausal vaginal bleeding and a mass in the apex of the vagina. (*A*) Coronal T2-weighted MR imaging of the pelvis shows a mass in the apex of the vagina (*arrow*). (*B*) Axial FDG-PET/CT shows a hypermetabolic mass in the vagina with no evidence of hypermetabolic adenopathy. The patient was treated with targeted intensity modulated radiation therapy to the vagina (*arrow*).

detection of adenopathy does not change the overall clinical stage. However, studies have suggested that lymph node metastases indicate poor prognosis.[61] FDG imaging can therefore potentially provide a noninvasive method to diagnose lymph node metastases (**Fig. 4**). In patients with vaginal or cervical cancer who have suspected recurrence, FDG-PET has a sensitivity of 100% and specificity of 73% for detection of extrapelvic disease after pelvic radiation.[62]

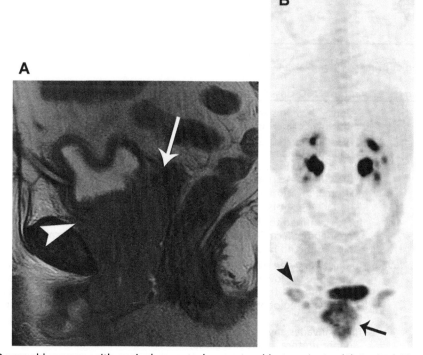

Fig. 4. A 53-year-old woman with vaginal cancer who was unable to urinate. (A) Sagittal T2-weighted MR imaging of the pelvis shows a mass in the anterior lip of the vagina (*arrow*) that encases the urethra (*arrowhead*). (*B*) Coronal FDG-PET MIP image shows a hypermetabolic mass in the vagina (*arrow*) and right inguinal adenopathy (*arrowhead*). There is no evidence of extrapelvic disease. The patient was treated with total pelvic radiation and adjuvant chemotherapy.

Therefore, FDG-PET can be used to identify patients who are candidates for pelvic exenteration for localized recurrence in the pelvis.

VULVAR CARCINOMA

Vulvar carcinomas are uncommon tumors accounting for 4% of gynecologic malignancies. About 3600 cases are diagnosed in the United States each year, with fewer than 1000 deaths.[7,63] Vulvar carcinoma usually occurs in women in the seventh decade of life but can be seen in younger women who have HPV. Most vulvar carcinomas are squamous cell cancers. Other rare malignancies are adenocarcinomas, melanoma, and sarcoma or basal cell carcinoma. These tumors are usually detected at early clinical stages without obvious metastases, and are staged according to the FIGO system (Table 3).[64] The standard treatment of invasive squamous cell carcinoma of the vulva is wide local reexcision and lymph node dissection. Typical patterns of spread include local invasion and lymphatic dissemination. The vulva primarily drains into inguinal lymph nodes ipsilateral to the primary tumor. If the tumor extends to the midline or the clitoris, both right and left inguinal lymph nodes are at risk and can be involved. Vulvar cancer can spread to pelvic lymph nodes, but as a rule only in association with inguinal node involvement.[65] At present there is no reliable noninvasive technique available to detect metastases. Inguinofemoral dissection is associated with significant morbidity. Lymph node metastases are an important prognostic factor in vulvar cancer. The incidence of nodal metastases in the groin increases with size and depth of invasion. Even superficial tumors of 5 mm or less can be associated with lymph node metastases in 20% of cases.[66] The presence of lymph node metastases decreased 5-year survival from 97% (stage I) to 50% (stage III).[64] Currently no reliable noninvasive technique can detect metastases, and inguinofemoral dissection is associated with significant morbidity.[67] Accurate preoperative staging may reduce the need for unnecessary lymphadenectomy resulting in a subsequent decrease in surgical morbidity.

Isosulfan blue dye and Tc 99m sulfur colloid have been used to map sentinel lymph nodes and provide a landmark for dissection.[68,69] However, this is less suitable in tumors located on the midline.[70] In this case identifying sentinel lymph nodes on one side does not preclude groin dissection on the other side. FDG-PET/CT may be helpful in such situations. MR imaging has also been used for the staging of

Table 3
FIGO staging of primary vulvar cancer

FIGO staging	Current FIGO classification	Treatment
Stage IA	Lesions ≤2 cm in size, confined to the vulva or perineum and with stromal invasion ≤1.0 mm, no nodal metastasis	Radiation versus surgery and groin lymph node dissection
Stage IB	Lesions ≤2 cm in size, confined to the vulva or perineum and with stromal invasion >1.0 mm, no nodal metastasis	
Stage II	Tumor confined to the vulva and/or perineum; >2 cm in greatest dimension; no nodal metastasis	Radical vulvectomy with bilateral inguinofemoral dissection and adjuvant radiation
Stage III	Tumor of any size with adjacent spread to the lower urethra and/or the vagina, or the anus and/or unilateral regional lymph node metastasis	Preoperative radiation, radical vulvectomy with bilateral inguinofemoral dissection and adjuvant chemoradiation
Stage IVA	Tumor invades any of the following: upper urethra, bladder mucosa, rectal mucosa, pelvic bone, and/or bilateral regional node metastases	
Stage IVB	Any distant metastasis including pelvic lymph nodes	Palliative chemotherapy

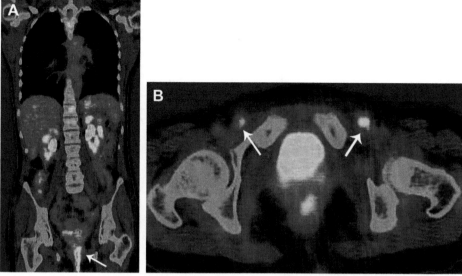

Fig. 5. A 37-year-old woman with 1.2-mm-deep vulvar cancer. (A) Coronal FDG-PET/CT shows a metabolically active mass in the vulva (arrow). (B) Axial FDG-PET/CT shows hypermetabolic lymph nodes (arrows), which were pathologically proved to be nonmalignant. The patient was treated with radiation.

vulvar cancer. Detection of lymph node metastases is largely based on the size and location of nodes. Malignancy is suspected in nodes that have a short-to-long-axis ratio of 0.75 or more. Using these criteria, the sensitivity and specificity of MR imaging for detecting lymph node metastases are 87% and 81%, respectively.[71]

The rationale for using FDG-PET/CT at our institution is that vulvar cancers have the same histology as squamous cell cancers of the cervix and are associated with the presence of HPV virus, and therefore FDG-PET/CT should perform in a similar manner. FDG imaging may be able to identify metastases to all lymph nodes in a single noninvasive examination (Figs. 5 and 6). One

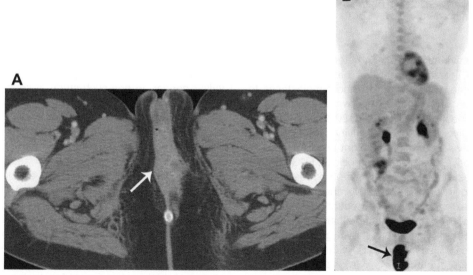

Fig. 6. A 45-year-old woman with locally advanced vulvar carcinoma. (A) Axial contrast-enhanced CT scan shows a large enhancing mass in the vulva (arrow). (B) Coronal FDG-PET MIP image shows intense tracer uptake in the primary tumor (arrow) with no evidence of hypermetabolic lymph nodes.

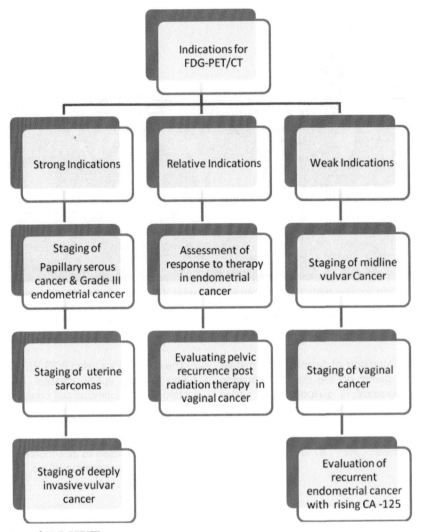

Fig. 7. Indications of FDG-PET/CT.

prospective surgical staging study has evaluated FDG-PET before surgery for patients with vulvar carcinoma, with respect to nodal metastases to the groin and reported an overall sensitivity of 80%, specificity 90%, PPV 80%, and NPV of 90%. Given the low sensitivity and high NPV, a negative scan result does not preclude surgical resection. Given the high specificity, FDG imaging identifies metastatic pelvic lymph nodes and can be used to plan preoperative chemoradiation or spare extensive groin dissection with patients being referred to treatment definitive chemoradiation, both of which have shown good pathologic response in some patients with an associated good clinical outcome.[72,73] In cases where FDG-PET identifies distant metastases, patients are exclusively treated with chemotherapy, as radiation has not been proved to improve survival.

PET using other radiolabeled amino acids such as [^{11}C]tyrosine are investigated for staging of vulvar cancer. In one such study, a sensitivity of 75% and specificity of 62% were reported for detecting inguinofemoral nodal metastases.[74]

SUMMARY

FDG-PET/CT has been widely evaluated in cervical and ovarian malignancies. The absolute and relative indications of FDG imaging in gynecologic malignancies other than those mentioned earlier are outlined in **Fig. 7**, and may change with future advances in technology and research. FDG-PET/CT has a limited role in the diagnosis of endometrial cancer, except for staging of papillary serous and grade III endometrial cancer, tumors with a high probability of distant metastatic dissemination. Similarly, FGD-PET/CT can be used in the staging of uterine sarcomas to prevent unnecessary procedures when distant metastases are present. FDG-PET/CT may be used in the detection of recurrent endometrial cancers in patients with increasing CA-125 values.

FDG-PET/CT has no role in diagnosing vaginal and vulvar cancers that are well seen on physical examination. However, it can be used in staging of deeply invasive vulvar tumors, which have a high preponderance of distant metastases. FDG-PET/CT may be helpful in indentifying metastatic lymph nodes in vaginal cancer, in locations dependent on the site of the primary tumor. FDG-PET/CT may also be helpful to detect recurrent vaginal cancer after therapy, and to identify candidates who may benefit from pelvic exenteration. The use of FDG-PET/CT in patients with vulvar cancer is undefined. Early studies suggest that it may be used to identify metastatic adenopathy.

REFERENCES

1. Pandit-Taskar N. Oncologic imaging in gynecologic malignancies. J Nucl Med 2005;46(11):1842–50.
2. Chao A, Chang TC, Ng KK, et al. 18F-FDG PET in the management of endometrial cancer. Eur J Nucl Med Mol Imaging 2006;33(1):36–44.
3. Kiesewetter DO, Kilbourn MR, Landvatter SW, et al. Preparation of four fluorine-18-labeled estrogens and their selective uptakes in target tissues of immature rats. J Nucl Med 1984;25(11):1212–21.
4. Mankoff DA, Tewson TJ, Eary JF. Analysis of blood clearance and labeled metabolites for the estrogen receptor tracer [F-18]-16 alpha-fluoroestradiol (FES). Nucl Med Biol 1997;24(4):341–8.
5. Lerman H, Metser U, Grisaru D, et al. Normal and abnormal 18F-FDG endometrial and ovarian uptake in pre- and postmenopausal patients: assessment by PET/CT. J Nucl Med 2004;45(2):266–71.
6. Horner MJ, Krapcho M, Neyman N, et al. Endometrial cancer and estrogen. SEER cancer statistics review [1975–2006]. Available at: http://seer.cancer.gov/statfacts/html/corp.html. Accessed January 25, 2010.
7. Jemal A, Siegel R, Ward E, et al. Cancer statistics, 2009. CA Cancer J Clin 2009;59(4):225–49.
8. Creasman WT, Kohler MF, Odicino F, et al. Prognosis of papillary serous, clear cell, and grade 3 stage I carcinoma of the endometrium. Gynecol Oncol 2004;95(3):593–6.
9. Creutzberg CL, van Putten WL, Koper PC, et al. Surgery and postoperative radiotherapy versus surgery alone for patients with stage-1 endometrial carcinoma: multicentre randomised trial. PORTEC Study Group. Post operative radiation therapy in endometrial carcinoma. Lancet 2000;355(9213):1404–11.
10. Benshushan A. Endometrial adenocarcinoma in young patients: evaluation and fertility-preserving treatment. Eur J Obstet Gynecol Reprod Biol 2004;117(2):132–7.
11. Hanf V, Gunthert AR, Emons G. Endometrial cancer. Onkologie 2003;26(5):429–36.
12. Chaudhry S, Reinhold C, Guermazi A, et al. Benign and malignant diseases of the endometrium. Top Magn Reson Imaging 2003;14(4):339–57.
13. Frei KA, Kinkel K, Bonel HM, et al. Prediction of deep myometrial invasion in patients with endometrial cancer: clinical utility of contrast-enhanced MR imaging-a meta-analysis and Bayesian analysis. Radiology 2000;216(2):444–9.
14. Duk JM, Aalders JG, Fleuren GJ, et al. CA 125: a useful marker in endometrial carcinoma. Am J Obstet Gynecol 1986;155(5):1097–102.
15. Han SS, Lee SH, Kim DH, et al. Evaluation of preoperative criteria used to predict lymph node metastasis in endometrial cancer. Acta Obstet Gynecol Scand 2010;89(2):168–74.
16. Tsujikawa T, Yoshida Y, Mori T, et al. Uterine tumors: pathophysiologic imaging with 16alpha-[18F]fluoro-17beta-estradiol and 18F fluorodeoxyglucose PET–initial experience. Radiology 2008;248(2):599–605.
17. Tsujikawa T, Yoshida Y, Kudo T, et al. Functional images reflect aggressiveness of endometrial carcinoma: estrogen receptor expression combined with 18F-FDG PET. J Nucl Med 2009;50(10):1598–604.
18. Torizuka T, Kanno T, Futatsubashi M, et al. Imaging of gynecologic tumors: comparison of (11)C-choline PET with (18)F-FDG PET. J Nucl Med 2003;44(7):1051–6.
19. Belhocine T, De Barsy C, Hustinx R, et al. Usefulness of (18)F-FDG PET in the post-therapy surveillance of endometrial carcinoma. Eur J Nucl Med Mol Imaging 2002;29(9):1132–9.
20. Liu Y. Benign ovarian and endometrial uptake on FDG PET-CT: patterns and pitfalls. Ann Nucl Med 2009;23(2):107–12.
21. Manfredi R, Mirk P, Maresca G, et al. Local-regional staging of endometrial carcinoma: role of MR imaging in surgical planning. Radiology 2004;231(2):372–8.
22. Manfredi R, Gui B, Maresca G, et al. Endometrial cancer: magnetic resonance imaging. Abdom Imaging 2005;30(5):626–36.
23. Petru E, Luck HJ, Stuart G, et al. Gynecologic Cancer Intergroup (GCIG) proposals for changes of the current FIGO staging system. Eur J Obstet Gynecol Reprod Biol 2009;143(2):69–74.
24. Suzuki R, Miyagi E, Takahashi N, et al. Validity of positron emission tomography using fluoro-2-deoxyglucose for the preoperative evaluation of

endometrial cancer. Int J Gynecol Cancer 2007; 17(4):890–6.

25. Kamura T, Tsukamoto N, Tsuruchi N, et al. Multivariate analysis of the histopathologic prognostic factors of cervical cancer in patients undergoing radical hysterectomy. Cancer 1992;69(1):181–6.

26. Kitajima K, Murakami K, Yamasaki E, et al. Accuracy of 18F-FDG PET/CT in detecting pelvic and para-aortic lymph node metastasis in patients with endometrial cancer. AJR Am J Roentgenol 2008;190(6): 1652–8.

27. Morrow CP, Bundy BN, Kurman RJ, et al. Relationship between surgical-pathological risk factors and outcome in clinical stage I and II carcinoma of the endometrium: a Gynecologic Oncology Group study. Gynecol Oncol 1991;40(1):55–65.

28. Irvin WP, Rice LW, Berkowitz RS. Advances in the management of endometrial adenocarcinoma. A review. J Reprod Med 2002;47(3):173–89 [discussion: 189–90].

29. Cherchi PL, Dessole S, Ruiu GA, et al. The value of serum CA 125 and association CA 125/CA 19-9 in endometrial carcinoma. Eur J Gynaecol Oncol 1999;20(4):315–7.

30. Saga T, Higashi T, Ishimori T, et al. Clinical value of FDG-PET in the follow up of post-operative patients with endometrial cancer. Ann Nucl Med 2003;17(3): 197–203.

31. Chung HH, Kang WJ, Kim JW, et al. The clinical impact of [(18)F]FDG PET/CT for the management of recurrent endometrial cancer: correlation with clinical and histological findings. Eur J Nucl Med Mol Imaging 2008;35(6):1081–8.

32. Park JY, Kim EN, Kim DY, et al. Clinical impact of positron emission tomography or positron emission tomography/computed tomography in the posttherapy surveillance of endometrial carcinoma: evaluation of 88 patients. Int J Gynecol Cancer 2008; 18(6):1332–8.

33. Sironi S, Picchio M, Landoni C, et al. Post-therapy surveillance of patients with uterine cancers: value of integrated FDG PET/CT in the detection of recurrence. Eur J Nucl Med Mol Imaging 2007;34(4):472–9.

34. Lin LL, Grigsby PW, Powell MA, et al. Definitive radiotherapy in the management of isolated vaginal recurrences of endometrial cancer. Int J Radiat Oncol Biol Phys 2005;63(2):500–4.

35. Brooks SE, Zhan M, Cote T, et al. Surveillance, epidemiology, and end results analysis of 2677 cases of uterine sarcoma 1989-1999. Gynecol Oncol 2004;93(1):204–8.

36. Inthasorn P, Carter J, Valmadre S, et al. Analysis of clinicopathologic factors in malignant mixed Mullerian tumors of the uterine corpus. Int J Gynecol Cancer 2002;12(4):348–53.

37. Yamada SD, Burger RA, Brewster WR, et al. Pathologic variables and adjuvant therapy as predictors of recurrence and survival for patients with surgically evaluated carcinosarcoma of the uterus. Cancer 2000;88(12):2782–6.

38. Major FJ, Blessing JA, Silverberg SG, et al. Prognostic factors in early-stage uterine sarcoma. A Gynecologic Oncology Group study. Cancer 1993; 71(4 Suppl):1702–9.

39. Sartori E, Bazzurini L, Gadducci A, et al. Carcinosarcoma of the uterus: a clinicopathological multicenter CTF study. Gynecol Oncol 1997;67(1):70–5.

40. McLeod AJ, Zornoza J, Shirkhoda A. Leiomyosarcoma: computed tomographic findings. Radiology 1984;152 (1):133–6.

41. Rha SE, Byun JY, Jung SE, et al. CT and MRI of uterine sarcomas and their mimickers. AJR Am J Roentgenol 2003;181(5):1369–74.

42. Umesaki N, Tanaka T, Miyama M, et al. Positron emission tomography with (18)F-fluorodeoxyglucose of uterine sarcoma: a comparison with magnetic resonance imaging and power Doppler imaging. Gynecol Oncol 2001;80(3):372–7.

43. Ho KC, Lai CH, Wu TI, et al. 18F-fluorodeoxyglucose positron emission tomography in uterine carcinosarcoma. Eur J Nucl Med Mol Imaging 2008;35(3): 484–92.

44. Sutton G, Brunetto VL, Kilgore L, et al. A phase III trial of ifosfamide with or without cisplatin in carcinosarcoma of the uterus: a Gynecologic Oncology Group Study. Gynecol Oncol 2000;79(2):147–53.

45. Kinkel K, Ariche M, Tardivon AA, et al. Differentiation between recurrent tumor and benign conditions after treatment of gynecologic pelvic carcinoma: value of dynamic contrast-enhanced subtraction MR imaging. Radiology 1997;204(1):55–63.

46. Connor JP, Andrews JI, Anderson B, et al. Computed tomography in endometrial carcinoma. Obstet Gynecol 2000;95(5):692–6.

47. Reed NS. The management of uterine sarcomas. Clin Oncol (R Coll Radiol) 2008;20(6):470–8.

48. Hornback NB, Omura G, Major FJ. Observations on the use of adjuvant radiation therapy in patients with stage I and II uterine sarcoma. Int J Radiat Oncol Biol Phys 1986;12(12):2127–30.

49. Murakami M, Tsukada H, Shida M, et al. Whole-body positron emission tomography with F-18 fluorodeoxyglucose for the detection of recurrence in uterine sarcomas. Int J Gynecol Cancer 2006;16(2):854–60.

50. Sung PL, Chen YJ, Liu RS, et al. Whole-body positron emission tomography with 18F-fluorodeoxyglucose is an effective method to detect extra-pelvic recurrence in uterine sarcomas. Eur J Gynaecol Oncol 2008;29(3):246–51.

51. Park JY, Kim EN, Kim DY, et al. Role of PET or PET/CT in the post-therapy surveillance of uterine sarcoma. Gynecol Oncol 2008;109(2):255–62.

52. Creasman WT. Vaginal cancers. Curr Opin Obstet Gynecol 2005;17(1):71–6.

53. Creasman WT, Phillips JL, Menck HR. The National Cancer Data Base report on cancer of the vagina. Cancer 1998;83(5):1033–40.

54. Herbst AL, Norusis MJ, Rosenow PJ, et al. An analysis of 346 cases of clear cell adenocarcinoma of the vagina and cervix with emphasis on recurrence and survival. Gynecol Oncol 1979;7(2):111–22.

55. Melnick S, Cole P, Anderson D, et al. Rates and risks of diethylstilbestrol-related clear-cell adenocarcinoma of the vagina and cervix. An update. N Engl J Med 1987;316(9):514–6.

56. Daling JR, Madeleine MM, Schwartz SM, et al. A population-based study of squamous cell vaginal cancer: HPV and cofactors. Gynecol Oncol 2002; 84(2):263–70.

57. Al-Kurdi M, Monaghan JM. Thirty-two years experience in management of primary tumours of the vagina. Br J Obstet Gynaecol 1981;88(11):1145–50.

58. Frank SJ, Jhingran A, Levenback C, et al. Definitive radiation therapy for squamous cell carcinoma of the vagina. Int J Radiat Oncol Biol Phys 2005;62(1):138–47.

59. Frank SJ, Deavers MT, Jhingran A, et al. Primary adenocarcinoma of the vagina not associated with diethylstilbestrol (DES) exposure. Gynecol Oncol 2007;105(2):470–4.

60. Lamoreaux WT, Grigsby PW, Dehdashti F, et al. FDG-PET evaluation of vaginal carcinoma. Int J Radiat Oncol Biol Phys 2005;62(3):733–7.

61. Pingley S, Shrivastava SK, Sarin R, et al. Primary carcinoma of the vagina: Tata Memorial Hospital experience. Int J Radiat Oncol Biol Phys 2000; 46(1):101–8.

62. Husain A, Akhurst T, Larson S, et al. A prospective study of the accuracy of 18Fluorodeoxyglucose positron emission tomography (18FDG PET) in identifying sites of metastasis prior to pelvic exenteration. Gynecol Oncol 2007;106(1):177–80.

63. Johann S, Klaeser B, Krause T, et al. Comparison of outcome and recurrence-free survival after sentinel lymph node biopsy and lymphadenectomy in vulvar cancer. Gynecol Oncol 2008;110(3):324–8.

64. Stehman FB, Look KY. Carcinoma of the vulva. Obstet Gynecol 2006;107(3):719–33.

65. Curry SL, Wharton JT, Rutledge F. Positive lymph nodes in vulvar squamous carcinoma. Gynecol Oncol 1980;9(1):63–7.

66. Sedlis A, Homesley H, Bundy BN, et al. Positive groin lymph nodes in superficial squamous cell vulvar cancer. A Gynecologic Oncology Group Study. Am J Obstet Gynecol 1987;156(5):1159–64.

67. Rouzier R, Haddad B, Dubernard G, et al. Inguinofemoral dissection for carcinoma of the vulva: effect of modifications of extent and technique on morbidity and survival. J Am Coll Surg 2003;196(3):442–50.

68. Radziszewski J, Kowalewska M, Jedrzejczak T, et al. The accuracy of the sentinel lymph node concept in early stage squamous cell vulvar carcinoma. Gynecol Oncol 2010;116(3):473–7.

69. Levenback C, Burke TW, Gershenson DM, et al. Intraoperative lymphatic mapping for vulvar cancer. Obstet Gynecol 1994;84(2):163–7.

70. Hampl M, Hantschmann P, Michels W, et al. Validation of the accuracy of the sentinel lymph node procedure in patients with vulvar cancer: results of a multicenter study in Germany. Gynecol Oncol 2008;111(2):282–8.

71. Kataoka MY, Sala E, Baldwin P, et al. The accuracy of magnetic resonance imaging in staging of vulvar cancer: a retrospective multi-centre study. Gynecol Oncol 2010;117(1):82–7.

72. Beriwal S, Coon D, Heron DE, et al. Preoperative intensity-modulated radiotherapy and chemotherapy for locally advanced vulvar carcinoma. Gynecol Oncol 2008;109(2):291–5.

73. Rogers LJ, Howard B, Van Wijk L, et al. Chemoradiation in advanced vulval carcinoma. Int J Gynecol Cancer 2009;19(4):745–51.

74. De Hullu JA, Pruim J, Que TH, et al. Noninvasive detection of inguinofemoral lymph node metastases in squamous cell cancer of the vulva by L-[1–11C]-tyrosine positron emission tomography. Int J Gynecol Cancer 1999;9(2):141–6.

PET and PET/CT Assessment of Gynecologic Malignancies: Beyond FDG

Sandip Basu, MBBS (Hons), DRM, DNB, MNAMS[a],
Thomas C. Kwee, MD[b], Abass Alavi, MD[c],*

KEYWORDS

- Gynecological malignancies • Cervical carcinoma
- Ovarian carcinoma • Endometrial carcinoma
- PET • Non-FDG

The literature on PET and PET/CT imaging using novel PET tracers in gynecologic malignancies has been relatively limited and restricted primarily to carcinoma of the cervix, ovary, and endometrium. These tracers have been investigated for their potential to overcome the shortcomings of fluorodeoxyglucose (FDG) imaging. The absence of significant renal excretion with some of the tracers is particularly advantageous, making them theoretically more suitable than FDG for disease evaluation in patients with this group of malignancies located mainly in the abdomenal-pelvic region. The non-FDG tracers that have been studied in these settings are ^{11}C-choline and ^{11}C-methionine for carcinoma of the cervix; ^{11}C-methionine for carcinoma of the ovary; and ^{11}C-choline, ^{11}C-methionine, and ^{11}F-fluoro-17-beta-estradiol (FES) for carcinoma of the en dometrium. ^{60}Cu-diacetyl-bis(N^4 methylthiosemi-carbazone) (ATSM) and ^{64}Cu-ATSM PET studies have been conducted on carcinoma of the cervix for assessment of the presence of tumor hypoxia. High ^{11}C-methionine uptake has been reported in primary cervical and endometrial carcinoma, with only modest uptake of this tracer also noted in the normal endometrium. Some reports have also indicated that this tracer may allow for the differential diagnosis between benign and malignant ovarian neoplasms, whereas others have suggested that the detection rate of microscopic peritoneal disease and iliac lymph node metastases using ^{11}C-methionine is suboptimal. ^{11}C-choline had an almost similar detection efficacy for primary gynecologic malignancies, with false-positive findings being observed in cases of atypical hyperplasia of the endometrium and pelvic inflammatory disease. ^{11}C-choline has been advocated by some as useful in improving the staging accuracy of MR imaging in patients with cervical and endometrial carcinoma. Preliminary data have shown that PET imaging with both FES and FDG could provide pathophysiologic information for the differential diagnosis and grading of uterine tumors. Pretherapy ^{60}Cu-ATSM PET has been predictive of outcome in patients with locally advanced cervical cancer. At present there are

[a] Radiation Medicine Centre (BARC), Tata Memorial Hospital Annexe, Parel, Mumbai 400012, India
[b] Department of Radiology, University Medical Center Utrecht, Utrecht, The Netherlands
[c] Division of Nuclear Medicine, Hospital of University of Pennsylvania, 3400 Spruce Street, Philadelphia, PA 19104, USA
* Corresponding author.
E-mail address: abass.alavi@uphs.upenn.edu

PET Clin 5 (2010) 477–482
doi:10.1016/j.cpet.2010.07.006

no clinical data on the application of non-FDG PET imaging in malignancies, such as in carcinoma of the vulva, vagina, and fallopian tube.

NON-FDG TRACERS IN CERVICAL CARCINOMA

Imaging using both ^{11}C-choline and ^{11}C-methionine have been evaluated in carcinoma of the cervix. Lapela and colleagues[1] imaged 14 patients with either cervical or endometrial carcinoma with ^{11}C-methionine PET. Absence of significant renal excretion with subsequent little or no radioactivity in the urinary bladder makes this tracer more suitable than FDG for evaluation of gynecologic malignancies. All primary tumors showed increased uptake, with a mean standardized uptake value (SUV) of 8.4 in the tumor versus a mean SUV of 4.6 for the normal endometrium. Moderately or poorly differentiated tumor showed greater uptake than well-differentiated tumor.

Torizuka and colleagues[2] compared FDG PET with ^{11}C-choline PET in 18 untreated patients with gynecologic malignancies. Although ^{11}C-choline detected the primary tumor in 16 of 18 patients compared with 14 of 18 with FDG, SUVs were lower for ^{11}C-choline. Furthermore, false-positive findings were observed in patients with atypical hyperplasia of the endometrium and pelvic inflammatory disease. Detection of microscopic peritoneal disease was limited. Iliac lymph node metastases were missed because of physiologic intestinal activity.

Sofue and colleagues[3] retrospectively assessed 22 patients with uterine carcinoma who underwent ^{11}C-choline PET/CT and pelvic MR imaging, including 11 patients with cervical carcinoma. The T stage was correctly classified by MR imaging alone in 6 of the 11 patients, by ^{11}C-choline PET/CT in an additional 3 patients, and by the combination of ^{11}C-choline PET/CT with MR imaging in 6 patients. The accuracy of N staging was 73% by MR imaging alone, 91% by ^{11}C-choline PET-/T alone, and 91% by the combination of ^{11}C-choline PET/CT and MR imaging. One patient had M1 disease with involvement of a para-aortic lymph node. The accuracy of M staging was 100% by ^{11}C-choline PET/CT plus MR imaging as well as by ^{11}C-choline PET/CT alone. After treatment, tumor size, volume, and SUV decreased in 5 of the 11 patients with cervical carcinoma. A significant correlation was found between the reduction rate of SUV and the reduction rate of the tumor volume.

In a prospective study by Lewis and colleagues,[4] 10 patients with cervical carcinoma underwent PET on separate days with [60]Cu-ATSM and ^{64}Cu-ATSM. The toxicology and pharmacologic data demonstrated that the formulation has an appropriate margin of safety for clinical use. In the patient study, the image quality obtained with ^{64}Cu-ATSM was better than that obtained from [60]Cu-ATSM because of lower noise. Otherwise, the pattern and magnitude of the [60]Cu-ATSM and ^{64}Cu-ATSM tumor uptake found separate studies performed 1 to 9 days apart were similar. ^{64}Cu-ATSM appears therefore to be a safe radiopharmaceutical that can be used to obtain high-quality images of tumor hypoxia in human cancers.

Grigsby and colleagues[5] prospectively investigated whether hypoxia-related molecular markers were associated with [60]Cu-ATSM PET imaging of tumor hypoxia in 15 patients with cervical cancer. Six patients had hypoxic tumors as determined by [60]Cu-ATSM, and 9 had nonhypoxic tumors. The 4-year overall survival estimates were 75% for patients with nonhypoxic tumors and 33% for those with hypoxic tumors ($P = .04$). Overexpression of vascular endothelial growth factor ($P = .13$), epidermal growth factor receptor ($P = .05$), carbonic anhydrase IX ($P = .02$), cyclooxygenase-2 ($P = .08$), and the presence of apoptosis ($P = .005$) occurred in patients with hypoxic tumors. Cox proportional hazards modeling demonstrated hypoxia as determined by [60]Cu-ATSM PET to be a significant independent predictor of tumor recurrence ($P = .0287$).

In a feasibility study, Dehdashti and colleagues[6] prospectively assessed whether pretherapy [60]Cu-ATSM PET could predict response to subsequent radio- and chemotherapy in 14 patients with locally advanced cervical carcinoma. All patients also underwent clinical PET with FDG before the institution of therapy. Tumor uptake of [60]Cu-ATSM was inversely related to progression-free and overall survival ($P = .0005$ and $P = .015$, respectively, as determined by the log-rank test). Also, the frequency of locoregional nodal metastases was greater in hypoxic tumors (tumor-to-muscle activity ratio [T/M] >3.5) than in normoxic tumors (T/M $\leq$3.5) ($P = .03$). FDG uptake in tumors did not correlate with [60]Cu-ATSM uptake ($r = 0.04$; $P = .80$) and no significant difference in FDG uptake between hypoxic and normoxic tumors were found. The same researchers reported similar results in a larger study that included 24 additional patients. In this prospective study,[7] tumor [60]Cu-ATSM uptake was inversely related to progression-free survival and cause-specific survival ($P = .0006$ and $P = .04$, respectively, log-rank test). The 3-year progression-free survival of patients with normoxic tumors was 71%, and that of patients with hypoxic tumors was 28% (P = .01). Again, FDG uptake in the primary tumor did not correlate with ^{60}Cu-ATSM uptake. There was no significant difference in FDG uptake between patients with hypoxic tumors and those with normoxic tumors (P = .9). Pretherapy ^{60}Cu-ATSM PET provides, therefore, clinically relevant information about tumor oxygenation that is predictive of outcome in patients with locally advanced cervical cancer.

PET WITH TRACERS OTHER THAN FDG FOR METABOLIC IMAGING OF OVARIAN TUMORS

^{11}C-methionine has been assessed for potential metabolic imaging of benign and malignant ovarian tumors. Lapela and colleagues[8] studied 4 patients with 1 or 2 benign ovarian tumors (endometriomas or cystadenomas), 2 patients with a tumor of borderline malignancy, and 7 patients with ovarian cancer using ^{11}C-methionine PET before laparotomy. CT or MR imaging was performed as a reference. Tracer uptake was quantified by SUVs and the kinetic influx constants (Ki values). Benign or borderline malignant tumors did not accumulate ^{11}C-methionine, whereas all carcinomas showed significant uptake. The mean SUV in the primary carcinoma was 7.0 ± 2.2 and the mean Ki ranged between 0.14 min^{-1}. The distribution of the tracer uptake was highly heterogeneous in 4 of the 6 tumors. The investigators concluded that ovarian cancer can be imaged with ^{11}C-methionine and PET, and that this method may be of value in the differential diagnosis between benign and malignant ovarian neoplasms but because of physiologic accumulations and methodological limitations, the value of ^{11}C-methionine PET in the staging of ovarian cancer appears to be limited.

PET WITH TRACERS OTHER THAN FDG IN ENDOMETRIAL CARCINOMA

The study by Lapela and colleagues[1] included patients with both cervical and endometrial carcinoma (8 patients). An increased uptake of ^{11}C-methionine was found in endometrial carcinoma,

with greater accumulation in particular in high-grade lesions. Histologically poorly differentiated (Grade III) or moderately differentiated (Grade II) endometrial cancer accumulated more ^{11}C-methionine than the well-differentiated (Grade I) subtype (P = .04 for the SUVs, and P = .05 for the Ki values). The investigators concluded that uterine carcinoma accumulated ^{11}C-methionine more than the normal endometrium.

Sofue and colleagues[3] retrospectively assessed 22 patients with uterine carcinoma who underwent ^{11}C-choline PET/CT and pelvic MR imaging, including 11 patients with corpus carcinoma (among which were 9 patients with endometrial carcinoma, 1 patient with carcinosarcoma, and 1 patient with serous adenocarcinoma). T stage was correctly classified by stand-alone MR imaging in 9 (82%) of these 11 patients, by ^{11}C-choline PET/CT alone in 5 patients (45%), and by ^{11}C-choline PET/CT and MR imaging in 10 patients (91%). One patient with corpus carcinoma who had developed a vaginal metastasis was understaged by MR imaging alone. In association with ^{11}C-choline PET/CT, which showed discrete uptakes in the corpus and vagina, this patient was subsequently correctly diagnosed as having a vaginal metastasis. Although this one patient was understaged by MR imaging alone, staging by ^{11}C-choline PET/CT alone or by ^{11}C-choline PET/CT plus MR imaging was correct. Three (27%) of the 11 patients had N1 disease. The accuracy of N staging was 64% by MR imaging alone, 82% by ^{11}C-choline PET/CT alone, and 100% by ^{11}C-choline PET/CT plus MR imaging.

All patients had M0 disease. The accuracy of M staging was 91% by ^{11}C-choline PET/CT plus MR imaging and 82% by ^{11}C-choline PET/CT alone. On the other hand, ^{11}C-choline PET/CT alone overstaged 2 patients with corpus carcinoma as having distant metastases and 1 patient was overstaged by ^{11}C-choline PET/CT plus MR imaging as having M1 disease.

In a study comprising 16 healthy female volunteers who underwent PET following the administration of ^{18}F-FES, Tsuchida and colleagues[9]

Table 1			
PET tracers other than FDG investigated for gynecologic malignancies in clinical studies			
Name of the Malignancy	**Name of the PET Tracers Investigated**		
Cervical carcinoma	^{11}C-choline, ^{11}C-methionine, ^{60}Cu-diacetyl-bis(N^4-methylthiosemicarbazone) (ATSM), and ^{64}Cu-ATSM		
Ovarian carcinoma	^{11}C-methionine		
Endometrial carcinoma	^{11}C-choline, ^{11}C-methionine, and ^{18}F-fluoro-17-beta-estradiol (FES)		

Table 2
Main findings of studies investigating non-FDG tracers in gynecologic malignancies (case reports excluded)

Reference(s)	Year(s)	Main Findings
1	1994	Uterine carcinoma accumulates ^{11}C-methionine more than the normal endometrium; moderately or poorly differentiated tumor shows greater uptake than well-differentiated tumor
8	1995	Ovarian cancer can be imaged with ^{11}C-methionine PET
6,7	2003, 2008	Pretherapy [60]Cu-ATSM PET provides clinically relevant information about tumor oxygenation, predictive of outcome in cervical cancer
2	2003	^{11}C-choline PET can be used for imaging of gynecologic tumors
9	2007	The change of estrogen receptor concentration relative to menstrual cycle as characterized by FES PET is consistent with reports that used an immunohistochemical technique
10,11	2007, 2008	First (case) reports showing the potential of FES PET and combined FES and FDG PET in the evaluation of endometrial tumors
5	2007	[60]Cu-ATSM hypoxia correlates with overexpression of vascular endothelial growth factor, epidermal growth factor receptor, carbonic anyhdrase IX, cyclo-oxygenase-2, increase in apoptosis, and a poor outcome
4	2008	[60]Cu-ATSM appears to be a safe radiopharmaceutical and provides high-quality images of tumor hypoxia in human cancers
13	2008	Estrogen receptor expression and glucose metabolism of uterine tumors measured by PET showed opposite tendencies; PET studies with both FES and FDG could provide pathophysiologic information for the differential diagnosis of uterine tumors
3	2009	The combination of ^{11}C-choline PET/CT and MR imaging increases accuracy of staging in uterine carcinoma
14	2009	Endometrial carcinoma reduces estrogen dependency with accelerated glucose metabolism as it progresses to a higher stage or grade

reported that the endometrial SUV was significantly higher in the proliferative as compared with the secretory phase (6.03 ± 1.05 vs 3.97 ± 1.29; $P = .022$). In contrast, there was no significant difference in myometrial SUV between these 2 phases. The investigators concluded that FES PET is a feasible, noninvasive method for characterizing changes of estrogen receptor (ER) concentration relative to the menstrual cycle.

The feasibility of combined FES and FDG PET scans for the differential diagnosis of endometrial tumors has been recently reported.[10,11] Yoshida and colleagues[10] investigated the value of FES PET vis-à-vis FDG PET and reported that FES imaging could potentially provide more useful information than FDG PET with respect to the efficacy of hormone therapy. ER expression measured by FES appears to be preserved in endometrial hyperplasia and reduced in endometrial carcinoma, which at the same time maintained accelerated glucose metabolism measured by FDG PET.

The binding affinity of FES is 6.3-fold higher for ERα than for ERβ; however, one must be aware that a negative FES study in endometrial hyperplasia can occur in patients on tamoxifen therapy, presumed to be primarily because of binding of ERs to tamoxifen or its metabolites.[11] Tamoxifen, in this setting, may act by 2 pathways: it can reduce ERα expression and also compete with FES for binding ERα. However, the second cause appears to be the major factor determining a negative FES PET in this group of patients. The half-life of tamoxifen is approximately 7 days in patients with breast cancer who are on chronic therapy[12] and hence should be stopped for several weeks before the administration of FES tracer doses for imaging in cases where this differential diagnosis is a relevant clinical question.

The utility of combined FES and FDG PET has subsequently been investigated in a larger series of patients.[13,14] Tsujikawa and colleagues[13] prospectively assessed the relationship between ER expression (FES PET) and glucose metabolism (FDG PET) in 38 patients with benign and malignant uterine tumors. Patients with endometrial carcinoma showed significantly greater mean SUV for FDG (9.6 ± 3.3) than for FES (3.8 ± 1.8) ($P<.005$). Patients with endometrial hyperplasia showed significantly higher mean SUV for FES (7.0 ± 2.9) than for FDG (1.7 ± 0.3) ($P<.05$). Patients with leiomyoma showed significantly higher mean SUV for FES (4.2 ± 2.4) than for FDG (2.2 ± 1.1) ($P<.005$), and patients with sarcoma showed opposite tendencies for tracer accumulation. Tracer uptake in patients with endometrial carcinoma was significantly higher

for FDG ($P<.001$) and significantly lower for FES ($P<.05$) when compared with values in patients with endometrial hyperplasia. On the other hand, patients with sarcoma showed a significantly higher uptake for FDG ($P<.005$) and a significantly lower uptake for FES compared with patients with leiomyoma. The investigators of this study concluded that ER expression and glucose metabolism of uterine tumors measured by PET using the 2 different tracers exhibit opposite trends and could therefore provide pathophysiologic information for the differential diagnosis of uterine tumors.

Tsujikawa and colleagues[14] also investigated whether FES and FDG PET reflect clinicopathologic features in patients with endometrial tumors in 22 patients with endometrial adenocarcinoma and 9 with endometrial hyperplasia who underwent both studies. Although the SUV for FDG was significantly lower in endometrial hyperplasia than in carcinoma, a significant difference between high-risk (International Federation of Gynecology and Obstetrics [FIGO] stage ≥Ic or histologic grade ≥2) and low-risk carcinoma (FIGO stage ≤Ib and grade 1) was observed only in SUV for FES. High-risk carcinoma showed a significantly greater FDG-to-FES ratio (3.6 ± 2.1) than did low-risk carcinoma (1.3 ± 0.5; $P<.01$) and hyperplasia (0.3 ± 0.1; $P<.005$). Low-risk carcinoma showed a significantly higher FDG-to-FES ratio than hyperplasia ($P<.0001$). In the receiver operating characteristic (ROC) analysis, the most accurate diagnostic PET parameter for predicting high- and low-risk carcinoma was the FDG-to-FES ratio and determined the optimal cut-off value of 2.0, which resulted in 73% sensitivity, 100% specificity, and 86% accuracy, higher than the 77% accuracy for MR imaging. The investigators concluded that endometrial carcinoma reduces estrogen dependency with accelerated glucose metabolism as it progresses to a higher stage or grade. The FDG-to-FES ratio is considered the most informative index reflecting tumor aggressiveness and it is suggested that it will be useful in the noninvasive diagnosis and clinical decision-making process for the most appropriate therapeutic strategy in patients with endometrial carcinoma.

SUMMARY

A number of non-FDG tracers have been investigated in gynecologic malignancies (**Tables 1** and **2**). The body of data regarding the clinical applications of newer PET tracers in gynecologic malignancies is limited, although several (feasibility) studies have shown their potential for tumor differentiation, grading, staging, and predicting outcome. Combined

PET/CT holds great potential in this setting because of its ability to localize lesions and it is possible that the combined use of these newer PET tracers and PET/CT imaging will enhance their use in this group of tumors.

REFERENCES

1. Lapela M, Leskinen-Kallio S, Varpula M, et al. Imaging of uterine carcinoma by carbon-11-methionine and PET. J Nucl Med 1994;35(10):1618–23.
2. Torizuka T, Kanno T, Futatsubashi M, et al. Imaging of gynecologic tumors: comparison of (11)C-choline PET with (18)F-FDG PET. J Nucl Med 2003;44(7):1051–6.
3. Sofue K, Tateishi U, Sawada M, et al. Role of carbon-11 choline PET/CT in the management of uterine carcinoma: initial experience. Ann Nucl Med 2009;23(3):235–43.
4. Lewis JS, Laforest R, Dehdashti F, et al. An imaging comparison of 64Cu-ATSM and 60Cu-ATSM in cancer of the uterine cervix. J Nucl Med 2008;49(7):1177–82.
5. Grigsby PW, Malyapa RS, Higashikubo R, et al. Comparison of molecular markers of hypoxia and imaging with (60)Cu-ATSM in cancer of the uterine cervix. Mol Imag Biol 2007;9(5):278–83.
6. Dehdashti F, Grigsby PW, Mintun MA, et al. Assessing tumor hypoxia in cervical cancer by positron emission tomography with 60Cu-ATSM: relationship to therapeutic response—a preliminary report. Int J Radiat Oncol Biol Phys 2003;55(5):1233–8.
7. Dehdashti F, Grigsby PW, Lewis JS, et al. Assessing tumor hypoxia in cervical cancer by PET with 60Cu-labeled diacetyl-bis(N4-methylthiosemicarbazone). J Nucl Med 2008;49(2):201–5.
8. Lapela M, Leskinen-Kallio S, Varpula M, et al. Metabolic imaging of ovarian tumors with carbon-11-methionine: a PET study. J Nucl Med 1995;36(12):2196–200.
9. Tsuchida T, Okazawa H, Mori T, et al. In vivo imaging of estrogen receptor concentration in the endometrium and myometrium using FES PET—influence of menstrual cycle and endogenous estrogen level. Nucl Med Biol 2007;34(2):205–10.
10. Yoshida Y, Kurokawa T, Sawamura Y, et al. The positron emission tomography with F18 17beta-estradiol has the potential to benefit diagnosis and treatment of endometrial cancer. Gynecol Oncol 2007;104(3):764–6.
11. Tsujikawa T, Okazawa H, Yoshida Y, et al. Distinctive FDG and FES accumulation pattern of two tamoxifen-treated patients with endometrial hyperplasia. Ann Nucl Med 2008;22(1):73–7.
12. Fabian C, Sternson L, El-Serafi M, et al. Clinical pharmacology of tamoxifen in patients with breast cancer: correlation with clinical data. Cancer 1981;48(4):876–82.
13. Tsujikawa T, Yoshida Y, Mori T, et al. Uterine tumors: pathophysiologic imaging with 16alpha-[18F]fluoro-17beta-estradiol and 18F fluorodeoxyglucose PET—initial experience. Radiology 2008;248(2):599–605.
14. Tsujikawa T, Yoshida Y, Kudo T, et al. Functional images reflect aggressiveness of endometrial carcinoma: estrogen receptor expression combined with 18F-FDG PET. J Nucl Med 2009;50(10):1598–604.

Index

Note: Page numbers of article titles are in **boldface** type.

PET Clin 5 (2010) 483–484
doi:10.1016/S1556-8598(10)00114-8
1556-8598/10/$ – see front matter © 2010 Elsevier Inc. All rights reserved.

pet.theclinics.com

Printed and bound by CPI Group (UK) Ltd, Croydon, CR0 4YY

03/10/2024

01040358-0015